Praise for *Entertaining Cancer*

T0247426

I read this book in one sitting! It is
subject and demystifying in its impact. Devamitra cap—
optically in one's mind and poetically, 'Life is gossamer at the
mercy of shifting winds.' It has real whimsical charm. I hope it
is read by many, especially men. – **Corrine Bougaard**, Founder,
Artistic Director and Producer, Union Dance

Devamitra has written a compelling book about his cancer
journey that straddles a wide range of emotions: gruelling,
funny, poignant and uplifting. As a reader you are drawn
into his world as he undergoes particularly challenging cancer
treatment, whilst always maintaining a uniquely wry, even
amused, perspective on life and death.

All the way through he reflects on what Buddhism has to
offer his predicament, and clearly the strength of his practice
helps him to not only navigate this journey with character, but
to emerge enriched. The timeless teachings of the Buddha are
truly tested in the fires of his experience, and the confidence and
faith he finds in these teachings can inspire confidence and faith
in all of us. – **Vidyamala Burch,** co-founder of Breathworks,
author of *Living Well with Pain and Illness* and *Mindfulness for
Health*

Entertaining Cancer: The Buddhist Way is a remarkable book –
honest, lucid, unflinching, funny and radical in its willingness
to confront the facts of life and death. Devamitra's book tells the
story of prostate cancer, and how his Buddhist practice met the

challenges of diagnosis and treatment, even how cancer led to the deepening of his practice and his love of life. *Entertaining Cancer: The Buddhist Way* is not just for those struggling with illness or the fear of death; anyone interested in how Buddhism can help us live with courage, wit and generosity will find answers in this book. – **Maitreyabandhu**, author of *Life with Full Attention* and *The Journey and the Guide*

Devamitra, a senior member of the Triratna Buddhist Order, provides a very entertaining memoir on his prostate cancer diagnosis and treatment. It is an acutely observed and often painful account of a long ordeal, yet one liberally laced with wit and irony, gratitude and compassion. He writes fluidly and candidly, revealing the frustrations, joys and contradictions of modern health care, with pithy and amusing sketches of the situations and personalities he encounters. Although the subject is serious, he writes with a light touch and always warmly.

Many changeable thoughts and feelings come with the almost uncountable succession of ills afforded by the treatment, in stark contrast with the trivial presenting symptom of his cancer. The narrative flows easily, revealing almost incidentally, to this reader, how life is on the 'other side' of the consulting desk; the interminable hours in the chemotherapy suite, holding a tight bladder under the 'Saturn' or 'Mars' radiation unit; and enduring the punishment of his legs, at one time becoming incessantly restless, another time lifeless with fatigue. There is systemic enervation that confines him to bed, a numbness that impairs finger function, the skin changes, fingernails and hair fall out and more. Yet consolation comes in the way of music and from the love and care of friends. Devamitra writes movingly of his appreciation for their help, his affection for them equal to his love for the Buddha's teaching and path, and how this savage trial provides opportunity for deep understanding of the impermanent and conditional nature of human life. He realizes how much he longs to live only for the Buddha's teaching and to communicate it, to reach out to those suffering and in need.

Whenever the time comes for the author to leave us, this heartfelt, humorous and insightful account will no doubt be his 'parting kiss'. – **Siladasa** (Dr Mark R. Newton, FRACP)

Quite often stories about cancer are framed in terms of a battle. This isn't always helpful, as it implies that disease progression means defeat or failure on the part of the sufferer. Devamitra frames his account with interweaving themes of struggle, victory and setback, yes, but also of calm and insight. He brings to the story his physicality as a serious, life-long swimmer; his variable energy levels from the disease and the treatment; the importance of friendship; and the impact of words spoken during consultations with his doctors, nurses and acupuncturist. We hear this story flavoured with his love of romantic poetry, his deep engagement with Buddhist teachings and practice, and his devotion to his teacher.

I got to know Devamitra well in 1978, when he led the Buddhist retreat during which I joined the Triratna Buddhist Order. Our lives have intertwined since then in many ways, no doubt with some disagreements along the way! What a pleasure to read this book and get closer to the man and his wry, entertaining but deep reflections on life, cancer and everything. – **William Stones,** Professor of Obstetrics and Gynaecology and researcher in global health

Who would have thought that having cancer could be so instructive, and at times so amusing? Devamitra writes of his experiences with a style unique to him: beautifully crafted, engaging, witty, poignant, reflective and always disarmingly honest. If you have not had cancer you will surely understand what it means from reading this book. And if you have it now you will find a companion here who has faced with courage and clarity the terrors and indignities of this great test of character. Devamitra faces his test as a Buddhist, but he wears his Buddhism lightly, even though it is Buddhism that guides him through it. For him Buddhism is simply the truth about life, not a set of dogmatic beliefs, and so his writing is relevant whether or not you are a Buddhist. I recommend this book very highly. – **Subhuti,** author of *Mind in Harmony*

DEVAMITRA

ENTERTAINING CANCER

THE BUDDHIST WAY

Windhorse Publications
38 Newmarket Road
Cambridge CB5 8DT
info@windhorsepublications.com
windhorsepublications.com

Cover design by Dhammarati
Cover image by Joseph Matten, @humansbeing__

Typesetting and layout Tarajyoti

British Library Cataloguing in Publication Data:

A catalogue record for this book is available from
the British Library.

ISBN 978-1-911407-88-1

Contents

Author's Acknowledgements

Writers are rarely, if ever, the best judges of their own work and I am certainly no exception. My whimsical digressions can cause me to lose my own plot; worse still, my sometimes arcane sense of humour can baffle rather than amuse. Fortunately, my dear friend Sthiramanas (who appears in this account as Gus Miller) was at hand to call me to heel and keep me on the straight and narrative path. He generously applied his considerable dramaturgical skills to everything contained within these pages, helping me to bring order and sense where there was none, while firmly encouraging me to cut the many thousands of wayward words that escaped the story line, but that frequently were my favourite pieces. He has effectively been my editor and I am deeply grateful for all his help.

My heartfelt thanks and gratitude are due to Dhammamegha, together with the other members of the team and editorial board at Windhorse Publications, for all their enthusiasm, hard work, and support in bringing *Entertaining Cancer* to publication.

I owe particular thanks to Dhammarati for agreeing to

design the cover of this book despite having no recollection of having offered to do so – hardly surprising, as it was not a promise he had actually made! His design is the happy consequence of an amusing miscommunication, and I am therefore all the more obliged to him for his excellent work.

I am also indebted to Joe Matten for the arresting portrait on the cover, which was taken in a shoot a few days before I commenced chemotherapy. It catches beautifully the mood of this testing period of my life and the spirit of my words. I am further beholden to Alex Estrella of Exposure Films for so freely offering his expertise to promote this book through film.

Publisher's Acknowledgements

Windhorse Publications wishes to gratefully acknowledge a grant from the Future Dharma Fund and the Triratna European Chairs' Assembly Fund towards the production of this book.

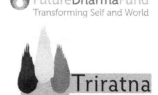

We also wish to acknowledge and thank the individual donors who gave to the book's production via our 'Sponsor-a-book' campaign.

Prologue

Dress rehearsal

I was in the middle of a five-month stint in Nagpur, teaching Buddhism mostly to young Dalits (formerly 'untouchables' under the Hindu caste system) at Nagaloka – a large campus-like centre of the Triratna Buddhist Community. Swimming was my main way of keeping fit when in Nagpur, and it was after a session at the municipal pool that I first admitted to myself that the bleeding was now fairly constant. As always, I was reluctant to seek medical advice in India. I talked it over with a friend who urged me to see a local dermatologist.

'If it bleeds, malignancy must be there', Doctor said, looking at the lesion my arm had been hosting for over fifteen years. It was bigger now – much, much bigger.

'But it doesn't bleed much', I objected, referring to quantity.

'It's spreading', he retorted, rather testily. 'It needs to be removed. Get biopsy first.' In Nagpur? Today! My accompanying friend understood perfectly well that I would not agree to this and that a nerve would have been pressed, but we both felt I needed to do something.

*

Like many of my Western friends, I had a love–hate relationship with India. After my first visit in 1971, I swore never to return, but, because of the legacy of Dr B.R. Ambedkar, my work for the Dharma (the Buddha's teaching) has taken me back so many times I have lost count. Ambedkar was born an 'untouchable' and had been the first law minister after Indian independence from the British Empire. In 1956 he had converted to Buddhism to escape the terrible stigma of untouchability. During subsequent years, millions of Dalits had followed his example; a few hundred of them are members of the Triratna Buddhist Order, like me, and many of them are my friends.

I have visited India to teach most years since 1987 when I was introduced, before giving talks all over Bombay, as an ex-film star. Like any myth, if repeated often enough it becomes an accepted fact.

'What part did you play in *Spiderman?*' was a question I was asked several times by students at Nagaloka. No matter how many times I asserted to my young friends that I had been a theatre actor, not a film actor, I could not dispel the fiction. Still I would occasionally hear the word 'Spiderman' intermixed with Hindi when being proudly introduced to visiting friends or family. I was both amused and embarrassed, but also flattered.

Nowadays I always look forward to going to India, despite the many challenges that life there offers. Basic assumptions are frequently undermined, which can be quite unnerving when you are used to everything functioning as you expect: no power cuts, constant running water, everything in place as it should be. When performing such simple tasks as washing out a cafetière in a sink, for example, unwary foreigners don't expect to get wet feet. It is so easy to assume that there will be a pipe beneath the sink to carry away the grounds and dirty water to some invisible drain, leaving your feet pukka clean, pukka dry.

Even some Indians may become complacent, forgetting, in moments of spiritual blindness, that Reality constantly shifts and changes. Just because a particular sink benefited from such a pipe the last time you used it does not mean that it will still be there the next time you do; the same applies to urinals, as I had discovered at the Nagpur municipal swimming pool. Pipes have a habit of disappearing with alarming frequency in India at times when you least expect and may most need them.

*

Life is unpredictable anywhere in the world, but in India it can be so to a disturbing degree. Not that I was particularly troubled by vanishing pipes, but anything to do with health could quickly arouse the deepest insecurity, as on the present occasion.

After the consultation with the dermatologist, my mind had reacted with characteristic anxiety. It had happened so many times. Any suggestion of medical or dental treatment in India and it would flare up, latching onto the fear of inadequately sterilized, or even recycled, needles and other medical equipment. It seemed to be an automatic response over which, apparently, I had no control – something instinctual, a function of body more than mind. No amount of assurances of hygienic equipment could assuage it, even though I had once submitted to a gastroscopy in Pune.

It was always the same. For years, this stubborn blemish on my arm had served as an easy object for irrational fear to seize as opportunity arose, unwilling to release its grip, like a wild animal with food clamped between its jaws, pursued by its erstwhile companions.

I had grappled with this sudden (generally short-lived) anxiety on many occasions, but it had taken time and effort to gain the upper hand. And now it was back with a vengeance; it was vital that I keep the initiative and so I reflected: if my body wanted to turn malignant there was little I could do about it – however, I could do something about my mind. And I did. Reflecting in this way helped to disperse the fear, and I concluded that it was time to give this irrational response the death blow. I would have this unsightly thing removed – in India.

*

I phoned Jivak, a fellow Order member, who, like his wife Asmita, was a GP.

'Come to Pune', he said without hesitation; 'you can stay with us. I'll organize everything.' And he did. Even better, I was a patient with two very attentive carers, both well qualified for the task.

'It doesn't look bad to me', Jivak said when I arrived. Even so, he and Asmita took me that same evening to a dermatologist friend of theirs.

'It's still just a wart', the dermatologist confirmed, but all three agreed it should be excised.

'What about the discoloured skin?', Asmita asked.

'Oh, that's just caused by something he's put on it', he replied.

'But I've never put anything on it', I said. He didn't seem to hear, but Asmita quietly took note and had a word with the surgeon.

*

I might just as well have been entering a garage as I stepped out of the dark the following evening with Jivak and Asmita, into the empty space that served as the hospital entrance. Another of their friends, a man renowned for his 'steady hand', would be dispensing with the wart. We climbed the stairs to the first floor of the building, then pressed the doorbell of what appeared to be a very large apartment but was actually a small infirmary.

As I lay on the surgeon's table, Asmita's warm and lively presence helped to put me at ease while her jovial colleague removed a slice of my flesh. At first taciturn, he had sprung alarmingly to life once the knife was in his grip, then deftly removed the wart and the discoloured skin surrounding it; both skin and wart were dispatched to a local lab for biopsy. When he got the results, Jivak told me that the discoloured skin had harboured a basal cell carcinoma (BCC), but not all of the bad cells had been removed; a second excision was recommended by the pathologist.

BCCs are uncommon in India as Indians are better protected from the sun by their pigmented skin, and so lack of familiarity had perhaps misled the dermatologist. And so, I returned for a second round of minor surgery, ten days after the first. This time, instead of Asmita's cheerful presence the room was filled with the bawling of two women rising from the slum below. How did they manage to sustain that torrent of high-pitched abuse for so long? It was raging when I entered the room as it was when I left it, somewhat groggily, twenty minutes or so later. But it had served to distract me from the wielding of the knife.

I now had 'a one hundred percent cure', the surgeon promised me. That would be nice, but what in life is so certain? I pressed Jivak to ask him about payment, but the surgeon would hear nothing of it, insisting that it was a contribution to my work in India.

Although that work was very modest, it was evidently appreciated. But I was uneasy to be the beneficiary of the surgeon's generosity, and determined to pay the medical expenses for someone who otherwise would not have been able to afford the treatment they needed.

The carcinoma had deeply alarmed me at the time – so much so that I'm amused at myself in retrospect. But a BCC is not usually a dangerous cancer. Nonetheless, having had to work consistently on my mental states so many times helped to prepare me for what subsequently happened, enabling me to see through the absurdity of my reaction and honing my capacity to respond equanimously to something truly life-threatening.

Preview

That had been in December 2014. Six months later, I moved into Sukhavati, a men's residential Buddhist community above the London Buddhist Centre (LBC) in Bethnal Green. In August 2016, Gus Miller, a young theatre director who had joined us earlier in the year, asked me late one evening, 'Would you like to be in a play, Devamitra?' I was taken aback, as I had left the stage behind forty-three years earlier, although I had never quite got the theatre out of my blood.

'Are you being serious?' I asked, as I finished brushing my teeth, excited by the idea.

'Yes', he said with a grin.

'Then send me the script and I'll let you know.'

We began rehearsals in early September; I liked the play and was enjoying working with Gus and the two other actors, but, just before I left for the theatre one morning, I knew that I had a serious health issue. A little over two months later, on 16 November, I was diagnosed with a suspected cancer. It was a life-changing experience. How that happened – and what those changes were – is revealed in this book.

The cast... and audience

In what follows, I have explained a few Buddhist teachings as this is necessary for understanding my approach to life, sickness, and death. But this is not a book about Buddhism. It is about the positive impact of Buddhist training on my experience of cancer and its harsh treatments. I hope it will be a source of inspiration to all who read it, and that readers might forgive my irrepressible sense of humour, which often surfaces in the most unlikely and painful circumstances. I further hope that it will be of value not just to Buddhists, but to all who suffer from cancer, those who are dear to them, anyone for whom the word itself inspires horror, and those who treat it.

Buddhism is at the heart of my life and has been for almost half a century. I have been a member of the Triratna Buddhist Order since I was twenty-five and so, inevitably, my experience of cancer has been significantly influenced by the impact of Buddhist teaching and practice.

Throughout my narrative I use the word 'spiritual' – a word I have never liked, but it is difficult to find a suitable alternative. In my usage it refers to the whole process of the evolution of human consciousness from a state afflicted by negative emotions and ignorance to its gradual transformation into universal compassion and transcendental wisdom – the twin pillars of the Buddhist ideal of Enlightenment. This process is not, as in the case of biological evolution, unconscious and automatic, but requires conscious effort.

You will encounter many people in these pages who have unfamiliar names because, like me, they are ordained Buddhists. They are my friends and, with the exception of my Buddhist acupuncturist and friend Niccala, they are all fellow Order members whom I know only by their Buddhist names. You will also meet my teacher, Bhante, otherwise known as Urgyen Sangharakshita, the founder of Triratna. 'Bhante' is an honorific term used when addressing a Theravadin Buddhist monk that literally means 'Venerable Sir'. Within the Triratna community, although Sangharakshita was no longer a monk, many of us used this mode of address when we were with him, or when referring to him, as an expression both of respect and of affection. Fellow patients and those who treated me also appear in this narrative; I have given pseudonyms to them all.

1

Diagnosis

I know the colour of that blood; – it is arterial blood; – I cannot
be deceived in that colour; – that drop of blood is my death
warrant; – I must die.[1]

When I first saw it, my mind went straight to Keats. *He* had
spat blood from his lungs, but this bright spurt had gushed
out at the head of my urine. There was no mistaking it any
longer; that slightly muddy colour, which for weeks had
escaped at the beginning whenever I passed water, was
merely the harbinger of this vermilion rush.

I must have a kidney stone; I dared not think beyond
my first assumption. The doctor was doubtful, but I was
tested anyway. Negative. I reluctantly returned. Bladder
or prostate, she insisted; a blood sample was taken in order
to determine my prostatic specific antigen (PSA) level – a
key diagnostic test for prostate cancer; it was 43. Anything
above 4 – even only by half a point – was considered high.
She manually examined my prostate gland and found a
large, hard abnormality. She would refer me for 'suspected'
prostate cancer, she said, but her manner and tone told me
at once that she had no doubts – and that it was serious. She
would request an urgent hospital appointment for me. Her

emotional attitude had suddenly shifted to a professional cheeriness through which I could see as clearly as through glass. And I felt suddenly thrust into another world – one that separated me from others by a word.

I left the surgery and walked to the park. It seemed extraordinary that I should have cancer. True, my paternal grandmother had succumbed to breast cancer, but she was the only one on either side of my family known to have had cancer; I have never been a smoker and was never much of a drinker; I have had no alcohol for close on forty years; I have always kept very fit and in recent years have practised intermittent fasting; I have been a vegetarian, mostly at the vegan end of the spectrum, most of my life and latterly have been completely vegan. The known conditions most likely to give rise to cancer have been absent from my life and yet it had finally chosen me – perhaps as my companion to death.

I needed time to reflect. What was I to do with whatever span of life might remain? How and where should I die? Who should I tell and how should I inform them? … And, thank goodness, my mother was dead. I was not being callous. I would have been unable to bear her anxiety and would have felt obliged somehow to survive her. Now, at least, I was free to die – one blessing; and another – should it prove terminal, I would dodge the rigours of old age; yet another – my body was too old for my restless spirit and was giving way increasingly under its strain. Well, now I could get a new one – but I must retain the initiative, meet death halfway before embarking on the great adventure.

I told a few friends and the men I lived with that I probably had prostate cancer... Why did that gap always appear? I am still in their world and they are in mine, yet they seem to drift away like ghosts – but not completely; then they forget and come back.

A couple of days later, I was lost in thought about where to die while being driven to a weekend retreat at Vajrasana, the LBC's retreat centre in Suffolk: somewhere remote, lonely, and beautiful – the west coast of Scotland, perhaps. I want to die alone, outdoors, in contact with nature.

'What about old Order members, Devamitra?' The question jolted me from my reverie. I hadn't a clue what my young friends had been talking about.

'They must learn to become ghosts', I replied, saying the first thing that came into my head. Singhamanas was driving; Ruta laughed. I forget who had asked me. They all seemed nonplussed by my response, as indeed I was myself. Why did I say that? But the more I thought about it the more it made sense.

I shared a room with Singhamanas and another team member, but had nothing to do on the retreat other than just be there, hang out in the background, a barely perceptible, positive presence. Because of chronic back pain I missed most of the meditation sessions and just sat in the retreat lounge looking out across the fields, or talking with anyone who came and sat with me – team members or retreatants; there was a constant stream. Occasionally I was alone, free to delight in the shifting light of the autumnal landscape.

Erection?

A week or so later, a specialist urology nurse explained to me the sequence of tests I had to undergo to determine my diagnosis: MRI scan, bone scan, and then a biopsy all within two weeks. The bone scan would determine whether or not the cancer had spread to other parts of my body.

The word 'suspected' was not part of her vocabulary, but they would only know for certain after the biopsy; then they could work out a treatment plan depending on the kind of tumour I had. Yes, my PSA level was very high, but not astronomical – it can hit the thousands. Surgery? Apparently, I would no longer be able to have an erection if I chose that route. 'That wouldn't trouble me.'

'Do you find it difficult getting an erection?'

'Well… it doesn't happen very often… but if I made an effort I'm sure there would be a response… I am an old man, you know.'

'Oh, no! You're young to have this.' *This* – no uncertainty that I have *this*.

'We'll need another blood test.' She glanced at my panier bag, frowning slightly. 'Did you cycle here?'

'Of course.'

'Do you realize that cycling pushes up your PSA because of the pressure the seat puts on the gland?' No, I did not. But it made no real difference because it would not push it up to 43; still, there could be slight inaccuracies in my results, including for the test I was about to have.

'You seem remarkably unfazed by all this.'

'Well, you haven't issued me with a death warrant yet', I replied, thinking once more of Keats.

'Oh, I don't think this is going to kill you!' She told me I could call her any time and gave me her mobile number. 'And don't cycle in for the biopsy. Probably best to keep off your bike for a few days afterwards, as well.'

Biopsy

While I was waiting at the hospital for the biopsy, one of the registrars approached me and asked if I would be willing to give a blood sample, together with my consent for the use of my medical record, for research purposes. They were hoping to find ways of identifying more accurately those who needed a biopsy.

I was somewhat reluctant to give them yet more of my blood, mainly because my two previous samples had been taken clumsily. (They seem to be forever after it; are they feeding pet vampires on the quiet?) He kindly took me to a phlebotomist who, he insisted, would be gentle – as indeed she was.

I'm glad that I agreed. The biopsy was excruciating; the fewer chaps who have to undergo it, the better. (The urologist only referred to men as chaps.) He gave me two injections of local anaesthetic directly into the prostate gland, then took twelve samples from it. It felt as if he was using a staple gun somewhere in my nether regions, stapling a chap back together. He rambled on, 'Not long ago they didn't give chaps anaesthetic for this procedure.' I cannot imagine how horrible that would have been for the chaps subjected to it.

The MRI scan had revealed a large growth covering most of my prostate and, just outside it, there were two enlarged lymph nodes looking 'highly suspicious'. (Internal terrorists perhaps? Or did he say nymph modes – that sounds more like my kind of thing.) But is it cancer? 'Highly likely.' (Why is he so cautious with his words? He knows perfectly well I've got cancer.) However, the bone scan had proved negative; there were no indications of cancer having spread elsewhere. But most alarming was the amount of blood that came out in my urine over the subsequent forty-eight hours. 'Most chaps find that it stops after a couple of days', but some of mine was still trickling out three weeks later.

The biopsy results would be ready in two weeks, but the consultant urologist was on annual leave. Consequently, I had to wait four weeks for an appointment. The nurse arranged a separate appointment so that I could be told the results, but, as this would not move things forward in any way, I cancelled it. I wanted to get away in time for the LBC's winter retreat in Herefordshire, and I did not want to think any more about cancer until I returned to the hospital.

Several people told me that prostate cancer was treatable and that most old men die *with* it, but not *of* it. 'It won't kill you' was something of a jocular refrain. And yet I knew that that was not entirely true, and it seemed to be at odds with the urgency with which my case was being treated.

Bhante

The retreat was a welcome change from visits to hospitals and their associated concerns. I really was able to leave it all behind, apart from the occasional butterfly stirring briefly in my stomach, but I was careful not to allow any to alight.

I had been hoping to see Bhante, but unfortunately when I arrived he was in hospital suffering from pneumonia and so I assumed that a meeting would not be possible. However, he was discharged just before the end of the retreat and, the day after his return, we met. He looked so weak and tired I dared not stay more than a few minutes; nonetheless, we were pleased to see each other.

He was then in his nineties, having just had a brush with death, and I wondered if I would ever see him again. He was twenty-three years my senior and I had always assumed that he would die before me, but that assumption was now rocking on its foundations. We had known each other for well over forty years and had quickly become friends after our first meeting. I knew that Buddhism stressed the importance of a teacher, but I had not properly understood why. One cannot truly learn the Dharma from books alone; one needs to absorb it from an experienced practitioner who not only understands the letter of the teaching, but has caught its spirit, otherwise it is easy to misunderstand and be led astray. It cannot be learned online; human contact is vital. Bhante had his own teachers, and they had theirs in a lineage ultimately leading back to the Buddha.

It had taken me quite a while to realize that Bhante was not just my friend, but also my teacher. I had responded immediately to his warmth and was fascinated by his extraordinary erudition. The breadth of his knowledge of the entire Buddhist tradition was equally matched by the amplitude of his comprehension of Western culture – its history, religion, philosophy, art, and literature. But what was most remarkable was that this breadth was complemented by an equivalent depth of understanding.

I had worked for him, worked with him, and lived with him for much of my life. And once more we were together, but this meeting, perhaps informed by a mutual sense of our own mortality, had particular poignancy. He mused with me about my health.

'You have done everything right and yet this has happened', he said. 'I sometimes think there is an element of luck in life… You remember how Napoleon chose his generals.' (Foolishly I had forgotten, but did not let on… or perhaps I had never known in the first place.) 'Before appointing them, he would ask, "Are they lucky?"' That was all, apparently. However, I do not consider myself to have been anything but lucky throughout my life, even now. I feel I have been blessed and, as I made clear to Bhante, that blessing had come directly from him – whatever his faults might be. My cancer is simply one of life's dirty little tricks. It keeps me on my toes lest I become complacent.

Confirmation

A few days after the retreat I was back at the hospital for the biopsy results. A young woman came through the swing doors and called out my name. I stepped forward.

'Hello', she said, before conducting me to her consulting room. Seemingly she was in charge of my case.

'Oh, I was expecting to see Mr Jones', I said.

'No. He's a urologist. I'm an oncologist.'

'I see', I said, immediately understanding the implication. 'So, you are going to confirm that I have prostate cancer.' My response seemed to throw her; she hesitated before replying.

'Well… yes, but you are a few steps ahead of me.' Moments later I was sitting opposite her in a windowless room as she explained that there was a spectrum of prostate cancer from mild to aggressive, and that mine was towards the aggressive end. My treatment would begin immediately with leuprorelin (hormone therapy), which would continue for three years. In case I should be in any doubt, she said, 'You have a serious disease.' My conviction too – and then, 'Are you able to have erections?' Gosh. The women in this department seem obsessed.

'I believe so. I mean, I don't exactly try… It's an embarrassing question.'

'Not for me. I ask it of men forty times a day.' Really?

(I could imagine my mother's response in her Teesside accent, 'Ee, whatever next, lad?')

*

The next step was a positron emission tomography (PET) scan to see whether or not there was any 'activity' elsewhere in my body.

'I do expect both lymph nodes to light up', she warned, 'but I will be surprised if anything else does', she continued, more reassuringly. 'However, we need to be sure about that before we can move on to the next phase of treatment. If the scan highlights nothing new, this will further confirm that the cancer is still contained within the pelvis and is therefore curable.' I would then receive six infusions of chemotherapy, at intervals of three weeks, followed later in the year by eight weeks of daily radiotherapy. 'You might like to read these.' It was information on chemotherapy and 'locally advanced prostate cancer'.

'Thanks, but I probably won't bother', I said, taking them. She then gave me a prescription for the hormone therapy. I was to begin with a short course of tablets to prevent a testosterone flare. This would then be followed about a week later by a first injection of leuprorelin, to be given at my GP's surgery and repeated every twelve weeks.

Leuprorelin would inhibit the production of testosterone, which generates the prostate cancer cells. There might be side effects, she pointed out with a hint of amusement, 'Similar to those of a postmenopausal woman: mood swings, hot flushes… You may also develop some tissue.'

'You mean man boobs?' I asked, slightly alarmed at what this might mean at the swimming pool.

'Possibly.' Crikey. We said goodbye and I went to collect my prescription.

As I was leaving the hospital, I recognized Jayamitra, one of my fellow Order members, on his way in.

'Devamitra! Bless you! What are you doing here?' I told him. 'That's what I've got.' Thursdays seem to be the day for prostate patients. Unfortunately, in his case the cancer had spread into his bones, meaning that it was terminal. The first indication of anything wrong had been back pain from a tumour that had spread there, by which time it was already incurable.

I felt grateful for the flood of vermilion that had fled with my urine, months before. It was not yet a death warrant, but a warning that I had heeded. I had had no other symptoms. How else could I have known?

Now that the cancer was confirmed, I needed to reflect further. I must not become complacent and assume that the PET scan would be clear. Milarepa, a great medieval Tibetan teacher and poet, warns constantly against hope and fear;[2] the English poet Shelley speaks of 'Hope and despair, The torturers'.[3] Hope often arises out of fear, but, when it fails, despair frequently displaces it. I did not wish to indulge hopes that may turn traitor. Resisting the temptation of hope was a growing point, an opportunity for me to rise above and beyond the reach of its unwholesome companions.

The real battle I faced was not with my body, but within my mind. I had understood this the moment I walked out of my GP's surgery with 'suspected' prostate cancer. What

I feared most was not death or pain, but loss of mental equilibrium. So far, I had succeeded, but there were tougher tests ahead. One came from an unexpected quarter.

Informing others

As there was no longer even a theoretical doubt that I had cancer, I wanted more of my friends to know and I decided to email some of them. The responses I received, as you would expect, were all concerned and sympathetic, but, in some cases, there was an element of anxiety – not mine, but theirs – and this could be quite difficult. They seemed to need to talk about it in a way that I did not. I simply wanted them to know and would have preferred to leave it at that, as I did not want cancer, or talking about it, to dominate my life more than was absolutely necessary. Naively, it had not occurred to me that some of them might need to talk with me about it more than I cared to do so. Occasionally I found myself in the anomalous position of having to reassure them about cancer – as if I was helping them to deal with their own fears.

If one of my friends was anxious, I could react to their anxiety with my own. Negative emotions can be contagious. When this first happened, I was rather thrown and asked myself why I had suddenly become anxious. As I reflected, it became clear that it was not *my* anxiety but theirs, and I needed to respond with positive emotion – patience, sympathy, or perhaps even compassion. From a Buddhist point of view, these positive emotions are all simply manifestations, varying in tone according to context, of the fundamental Buddhist virtue of metta, or universal loving kindliness.

Something similar happened when I received a letter from my GP's surgery inviting me to make an appointment to talk about my care plan; the letter began with an expression of regret at the news of my 'serious diagnosis'. Suddenly there was a butterfly in my stomach. I have never been a violent man, but I am at ease with the more forceful elements inherent in manhood and value them. Consequently, consistent with my aggressive character, I gave this flutterer the short shrift it deserved: 'Damn it! Leave me alone.' And it left me in peace. Such an approach may not work for everyone, but I have always been attracted by the heroic dimension of the Buddha's character and teaching, and have sought to emulate it.

I crumpled the letter and cast it away as if it were contagion. Although well-intended and clearly meant to be supportive, such comments can be counterproductive. Fundamentally I felt upbeat about my diagnosis. I regarded it as a challenge – not one that I would have chosen, but, since it was there, all I could do was meet it with the heroic spirit underlying the entire Buddhist tradition that was stirring within me. I must embrace it – even enjoy it for what it was. However, to do that I needed all the positive emotion that I could muster.

I made an appointment with an Order member who I knew was working as a locum at my surgery. I had noticed that it was she who had signed a prescription enabling me to have a hormone injection that I had had some trouble getting. This in turn had made it possible to receive the injection at an appointment I had made several days earlier with one of the surgery's nurses, which otherwise I would have had to miss.

When I met her she kindly asked if I was happy to talk about my 'care plan' with her, which of course I was. Not that there was much to discuss. I did not need a counsellor as I had an excellent community and many friends with whom I could talk about anything that troubled me (not that I could think of much, apart from dealing with the administrative inefficiencies of the NHS, wonderful though the NHS is in most other respects). The difficulty over my prescription had been caused by the hospital not properly requesting it of the surgery, apparently. I could well imagine, however, that the hospital would have had a different tale to tell.

Calvin's support

A few days later I phoned the urology nurse to let her know that I had had the leuprorelin injection, but there was something else bothering me. Ever since my GP had manually examined my prostate, I had been aware of discomfort both in my groin and further down. I had assumed that this was to do with my tumour, but I thought I had better ask the nurse as it was getting increasingly painful, and I mentioned rather gingerly that my right scrotum was so tender that even walking was painful.

'Oh, no!', she laughed, 'your tumour is inside your body, not your scrotum sac. Do you wear boxer shorts?' It is astonishing the intimate facts that one has to share with these ladies.

'Er, yes.'

'Try something more supportive – trunks, for example.'

'Ah, yes of course.' I thanked her for her suggestion, quickly concluded the call, lest we stumble into the erection question again, and promptly acted on her suggestion. Matters certainly improved with a little help from Calvin Klein.

Heightened awareness

Despite these minor concerns, in many respects my life had never been better. I rarely slipped into negative mental states, and even then, not for long. Many times, I walked around the lake at Victoria Park in East London appreciating its winter beauty, thrilling at the sudden flash of sunlight on a cormorant's wings or the brilliant green of the parakeets, the subtle winter colours adorning the trees highlighted by the sun's lateral rays.

No doubt this was all heightened by my medical issue, and I am grateful to the cancer for that. It is not that this was new, but I felt it yet more vibrantly and I have no doubt that that was due to my heightened sense of my own impermanence – precious moments that I must cherish fully, because I knew they would not, could not, last.

One such moment caught me unawares on a trip to Canterbury. Sitting alone, I was looking out of the train window at the rather dreary prospect as we sped by, when I felt overcome by a sense of detachment from the world and its problems. They were no longer mine to sort out. I was not being grandiose – of course, *I* cannot sort out the problems of the world – but somehow, they seemed not to be mine. It was not that I no longer cared, more that they seemed impersonal, beyond the purely personal, and as I continued to stare out of the window I was blessed by a deep tranquillity – the perfect mood to appreciate the seat of Anglicanism.

I had not been to Canterbury before and could not have imagined the impact that its wonderful cathedral would have on me. I have seen many of Europe's great churches, including plenty that are far more beautiful, but none that has affected me so powerfully. I cannot easily account for it, but I was swept away, as I wandered around, in awe of something I could not identify.

PET

Always at the back of my mind was the forthcoming PET scan; constantly, I reminded myself to resist expectations – to prepare myself for any outcome. This was a valuable tool – it was driving my heightened awareness of impermanence. I was beginning to think that the scan would find cancers elsewhere. Despite Calvin Klein, my nether regions were getting more painful, glands in my neck were swollen, and my upper rib cage had developed a rattle.

I should have gone to the GP, but figured that all would become clear with the scan and that therefore there was no need. I half expected to be told that I had not only prostate cancer, but also testicular and rattling-rib-cage cancer, with perhaps throat cancer thrown in as a bonus.

Finally, after further administrative problems, I had a date for the scan in the basement of the hospital and a week later I got the results. Oncology was running very late. As I entered the waiting area, I noticed Jayamitra sitting with his sister. However, rather ungenerously, I wanted to keep my mind focused and did not want to engage in conversation. Besides, I could not sit in those dreadful plastic chairs as they worsen my chronic back pain, and I always paced up and down when waiting, even if that meant for two-hour stretches or more, which it often did. But he had seen me and came over to say hello.

I was ashamed of my lack of friendliness, but was glad that he had given me the opportunity to make amends. Though I was sorry to hear that he was finding things increasingly difficult, both emotionally and physically, I was also suddenly confronted once more by my own predicament, as I was bracing myself to be told that I too might now be heading in that direction – at least physically if not emotionally.

Without thinking about it, I just said, 'Equilibrium of mind is more important than life', to which he quipped, 'Yeah! Equilibrium of mind is more important than life. Discuss!' I had meant to say that it was more important than death, because I had often dwelled on this thought. However, I enjoyed his jovial response. Soon afterwards he was called in for his appointment, and shortly after that I was called in for mine.

It took a while for the registrar to get on to the scan results, which she mentioned only in passing, casually indicating that nothing new had been revealed and that we could now get the chemotherapy organized. Somehow, she lost me and I could not quite believe what I thought I had just heard. Not wanting to be in any way impolite I did not wish to interrupt the discourse on chemotherapy, but I could not suppress the rising fit of giggles that disturbed it.

She was evidently taken aback by my strange, if not eccentric, response, but proceeded, 'You realize you will no longer be able to have children?'

I could contain myself no longer and laughed out loud, 'I'm sixty-eight, for heaven's sake. I'm an old man!'

'Oh, I don't know about that. One of my patients fathered a child at seventy-two', she replied, having caught my humour.

'And Picasso fathered one at eighty', I responded (this was not true, though I believed it at the time), 'and I'm no Picasso.' As we were veering dangerously close to the erection issue, I distracted her with a question about fasting. I had read about the research of Valter Longo, which suggested that fasting for a few days before and after chemotherapy both increased its effectiveness and diminished its side effects. I was keen to try it.

'One of my patients tried it and it just made her miserable', she objected with a hint of irritation. It seemed pointless to pursue the matter there and then.

Finally, we got down to dates for chemotherapy, which would start within a couple of weeks, after I had been briefed by a chemotherapy nurse.

Later, I discussed my thoughts of fasting with a nutritionist friend. Though he did not doubt that I could maintain positive mental states, he was concerned that four days of fasting, especially under the influence of chemotherapy, might make me feel faint. Thinking of the narrow, steep staircase that led down from my room, he asked, 'What if you fell and broke something? They would probably stop the chemotherapy then' – and so reluctantly I decided against it.

*

So, I did not have testicular cancer, but something was not right below. Two days later my right testicle had swollen to an alarming degree, looked very red, and was excruciatingly tender. As it was a Saturday morning I could not see a GP. Two of my community members urged me to go to A&E, so, resignedly, I walked bandy-legged (to minimize any contact between the top of my thigh and my swinging, overburdened scrotum sac) to my local hospital. Was I relieved to get there!

I was discharged two hours later with painkillers and antibiotics. I had had an infection resulting in epididymo-orchitis, which, I was informed, is an extremely painful condition. That was good to know; I felt less like a wimp. I was further assured that it had nothing to do with my cancer – although I suspect that there was a connection, as the whole episode was probably triggered by the manual examination of my prostate by the GP.

Consequently, for almost three months, I had tolerated the pain unnecessarily, understanding that cancer is a painful disease and having believed that the pain was from my tumour. One of the problems with cancer is that, if anything goes wrong, if you experience any pain, it is easy to assume that it is simply a symptom of the cancer itself.

2

Chemo Limbo – Impact

'Tell me one thing you would not be prepared to do on stage', the director said. I was one of the last to speak; everyone before me had mentioned something.

'I can't think of anything', I said. It was 1968 and I was an ambitious young actor. He paused and scrutinized me. Later, in rehearsals, he drove me into new terrain. And I loved it.

Reflecting back over my life I believe that my underlying attitude has remained the same. I have always tried to be open to new experience, but facing the challenges of a theatre director is not nearly so difficult as meeting those that life throws in our way and I am conscious of how many times I have failed. Nonetheless, it has been one of the guiding principles of my life. It keeps me alive, vital, and young at heart; it helps me not to settle down into habitual patterns; it is a reflex of the spirit of 'going forth'.

The principle of going forth has its origin in the Buddha's early life. According to his own account, while still young, he had reflected on the painful aspects of life – especially old age, sickness, and death – and sought liberation from them. Consequently, like many before him, he had gone forth from home in search of Truth, exchanging all the attachments of domesticity for the trials and adventures of a homeless wanderer. Eventually, he gained Enlightenment. But leaving home is just one manifestation of a deeper spiritual principle: the keenly felt urge to become a better and yet better human being, born of the understanding that this requires radical change. It is a transformation that is achieved gradually by constant effort to perceive and break down all psychological conditionings and habitual patterns of thought and behaviour, while displacing negative emotions with positive ones.

However, it is important to understand that pleasurable sensation and positive emotion do not always coincide. If I speak harshly to someone, I may enjoy an initial satisfaction, yet later I may regret my words. Regret is painful, but it is not a negative emotion, as it is a healthy response to the awareness that I have acted badly or, in Buddhist terms, unskilfully. That awareness, in combination with the unpleasant sensation of regret, spurs me to modify my behaviour and to expose and undermine the negative emotion that prompted it. Clearly, the pleasure of expressing my animosity is not positive, or skilful. Similarly, I may enjoy being tipsy, but intoxication is characterized by unawareness and is therefore unskilful from a Buddhist perspective.

Going forth is not something that is done only once. The intuition behind such a fundamental shift is the sense that there is much more to life than we generally perceive. This may be triggered by a sudden expansion of consciousness in response to some tragic experience; by the quickening of the imagination through the perception of beauty, whether in nature or in art (in the broadest sense); or when horizons unexpectedly widen and perhaps things are seen with greater lucidity. Most people have moments of this kind, but few are moved to act on them and go forth by reorienting their lives in accordance with their highest values.

I regarded my cancer treatment as a further opportunity to go forth. Chemotherapy was certainly going to be a new experience that I would not have chosen had I been ready to die but, if I wanted to live, I could not afford to spurn it. If I truly wanted to benefit from it, I must welcome it, just as I had welcomed the cancer.

I had no illusions; I knew that it would be a big challenge. It is difficult to imagine that anybody could enjoy its relentless rigour, but it is not my intention to give a blow-by-blow account of all the minor trials it threw in my face – that would make for tiresome writing and tedious reading. Nonetheless, in its unique way, I believe that the whole process was of significant spiritual benefit to me. It is hard to pinpoint anything in particular, as it is more to do with the overall impact of what, for me, was a kind of bardo. In the Tibetan tradition, a bardo is an intermediate state, generally referring to the period between the end of one life and the start of the next. However, the bardo of death is just one; meditation and the dream state are others.

First infusion

Just before I was about to start chemo, I was booked for a photo shoot in Birmingham and had been asked not to shave for the week before. It was not just welcome work; it was an opportunity to have evidence that I did once have long hair and that my beard could actually grow. One of the many shots taken that day appears on the front cover of this book.

The following week I received my first dose of docetaxel, the chemotherapy drug I had been prescribed. However, when I had arrived at the hospital I was told that my medication had not yet been prepared and that there would be a delay. I was finally called into the ward four hours later. Subsequently, I learned that such delays were not uncommon and that tensions between the nursing staff and 'pharmacy' were part of life on the ward.

A cannula was inserted into a vein on the back of my hand, which was then hooked up to a saline drip to flush my vein before and after the docetaxel, the whole procedure taking just under two hours. I was monitored closely by a nurse for the first few minutes in case there might be any adverse reaction to the drug; fortunately, there was none.

The ward, which was divided into five rooms, was at the top of the building and commanded an impressive view of the City. There were seven or eight treatment chairs in each room, and a quiet but friendly atmosphere pervaded the whole place. Quiet in my room, that is, apart from Teddy, the life and soul of the chemo party.

'She lives in the flat above mine', he explained, pointing to his already giggling wife, who sensed what was coming. 'Yer know what she does?', he continued with a big grin as he glanced round the room. 'She comes down in the middle of the night, creeps into me bedroom and holds a mirror over me mouth to see wevver I'm still breavin!' He grinned ironically while nodding his head at his amused listeners before resuming with greater emphasis. 'An' *then* coz she can't see anything', he proceeded, as an expression of amused disbelief swept across his face, 'she jabs me in the side of the 'ed like this', aiming two fingers at his temple, 'to see if I'm still alive. Then whoa! I wake up in a panic, me heart thumpin' away, wonderin' what the devil's goin' on.' Even the nurses had to pause in their work to control their laughter at this natural comedian. But later, when there were no visitors in the room, Teddy's mood swung in a different direction.

'The trouble with friends and relatives is they're so gloomy.' Then in a doleful voice of excessive solicitude, 'Ow are yer, dear? Are y' alright?' He shrugged and glanced upwards as if to ask: how do you respond to such inordinate concern? 'If yer not careful it can drag yer down. But I'm not gloomy, I'm hopeful. Where there's life, there's hope… In any case, I don't believe death is the end. I think we come back.'

'Me too', I chipped in.

'Do yer?'

'Sure, I'm a Buddhist.'

'Oh, y'are, are yer?' He paused, perhaps weighing me up. 'Have yer ever thought what yer'd like to come back as… have yer?', he continued, scrutinizing me further. '*I* have', he declared, with a hint of triumph, 'I wanna come back as *me*.'

'Don't worry about it, mate', I quipped, 'you probably will.' Not that I was suggesting that the man all his friends and family knew and loved would return recognizably, as Teddy.

Strictly speaking, I cannot say that I believe in rebirth, as I cannot recall any previous life, but the Buddhist explanation of continuous life, death, and rebirth makes sense to me. Consequently, my attitude to life, and therefore to cancer treatment, is strongly influenced by it, but the Buddhist teaching on rebirth can be easily misunderstood.

Imagine a candle slowly burning down until it is almost burned out. As it is in its final flickering and sputtering, the flame barely hanging on to the remnants of the wick, a breath of air carries it to another candle, standing just below, igniting it. This process then continues ad infinitum. The candle represents the body of an individual life, the flame its consciousness. Whereas each candle is unique and separate from all the others, the flame is seemingly the same; yet, like consciousness, it is shifting and changing constantly. Just as, within the flame, there is no constant or unchanging essence, there is no fixed element within consciousness, such as a soul or a self, and yet there is some sort of continuity from one life to the next – according to Buddhist tradition.

When someone dies, consciousness is separated from the physical body and eventually manifests in a suitable form. The main element determining that form will be the deep-seated, habitual mental states, positive or negative, that characterized the previous life. Thus, it is consciousness that determines form and not the reverse. If I constantly indulge feelings of resentment in this life, then that is likely to be a characteristic of the next; on the other hand, if I continuously cultivate generosity so that it becomes a habitual attitude of mind, that too will influence the character of the subsequent life.

Impact

Because of the pharmaceutical delay, I left the hospital too late to attend the team meeting before the Monday-night class at the LBC. I was due to give a talk that evening at the conclusion of a six-week course on the Dharma. As I did not know how many more such opportunities I might have, I was particularly keen to speak, but, more than that, I felt on fire – not with chemo, but with inspiration. I was in 'the crucial situation' – one in which I felt I had to grow or die, perhaps literally, but certainly metaphorically – and I wanted to take full advantage of that. By the time I began speaking, I was beginning to feel the effects of the chemo: fatigue in my legs and a slight headiness. Nonetheless, my words flowed freely and clearly.

Later that night, I suffered interminable hiccups and couldn't sleep. Consequently, I spent much of the night searching the internet for a cure. After several false starts I was reduced to sticking fingers in both my ears, while simultaneously holding my nostrils then breathing out before sipping water from a glass. Though it sounds absurd and probably looked even worse, because I was feeling desperate, I thus found an unlikely cure for my hiccups. Thank goodness nobody was watching, especially as I had succeeded finally only by using my swimmer's nose-clip to deal with the nostrils. I am already considered to be far more eccentric than I care for.

Forty-eight hours later the full force of the chemo began to plague and torment me. It was one of the worst nights I had under its influence: chronic toothache, sore gums, a mouth ulcer – and I forget what else – were just the backdrop to recurrent gastric reflux, which by 4am was so severe I called the chemo helpline.

When asked by the nurse if I had chest pain, naturally I said yes, which put an end to our conversation. 'Call an emergency ambulance immediately', she said. I insisted that it had nothing to do with my heart, but she kept repeating, 'Call an ambulance now!' I reluctantly gave way and awakened Vidyadaka, asking him to let in the ambulance crew. My call was made a priority so that, by the time he reached the front door, the paramedics were waiting – a short, plump, rather jolly woman and her taller, leaner, male sidekick.

I was greeted like a long-lost friend as Vidyadaka showed them into my room and they set to work and took charge of me with a will, sticking a variety of medical implements in my ear, in my mouth, on my finger, and on my chest.

Shortly afterwards, my phone rang. 'DID YOU CALL THAT AMBULANCE?' demanded the anxious-sounding chemo nurse.

My blood sugar was very low. 'Here, swallow this.' I sucked a sweet sticky substance from a tube as eagerly as an insatiable infant at its mother's breast and immediately I felt better. The sidekick was impressed as I had emptied the tube – a rare occurrence, apparently. 'Good, that's me sorted', I thought. But no; further tests were necessary in the ambulance. Damn it.

As we were about to leave the community, a figure emerged from the bathroom. 'Oooh another one!' chortled the paramedic as she fixed a startled male face with her eyes. (She'd obviously never been inside a men's community before and seemed genuinely thrilled.)

To my dismay, after several minutes in the ambulance, my new-found friends were dissatisfied with their tests and decided to speed me off to hospital before I had had a chance to let Vidyadaka know.

'Have you had a heart attack before?', asked the junior doctor examining me.

'Have I just had one now?', I asked, incredulously. She didn't reply but studied my notes more closely before seemingly confirming my own diagnosis of severe gastric reflux, advising me to double the dose of my normal medication. With that I was discharged – and it was still only 7am.

It was a fine, crisp winter morning and, as there were no buses in sight, I decided to walk back to the LBC. My legs were weak from the chemo, but I felt there was probably enough power in them to get me back. Walking slowly, it took me half an hour – twice as long as usual.

*

I had plenty to reflect on in the dazzling lateral light. Could I face another four months of this hell? Several people had warned me that chemo had a cumulative effect, implying that each cycle got tougher. (This was not my actual experience, by the way. As my treatment progressed, the side effects tended to settle down, although there was always something new.) If this was the price of life, was I really prepared to pay it? Would it not be better just to let nature take its course and let the tumour kill me?

When I finally reached the community, I kept my thoughts to myself. It was the only time I doubted that I could endure the impact of chemotherapy. My body seemed to be in total rebellion against it. I had had an extreme induction into the trials of chemo, but gradually all thoughts of discontinuing vanished.

Some of my friends seemed taken aback – even horrified – to hear that, after having disappeared in an ambulance to A&E, I had returned on foot, but I have always considered taxis an extravagance. Having been raised in Middlesbrough just after the Second World War when food, money, and fuel were scarce, I had the importance of frugality drummed into me and I have never lost the habit. Besides, enduring minor hardships makes you hardier – a necessary quality for one serious about practising the Dharma. Facing the realities of existence demands a mental toughness that many of us, living in the comfortable, wealthy world of Western democracies, lack.

Casualties

As best I could, I tried to maintain my normal routine – morning meditation, swimming, meeting people, writing, walking around the park, and classes in the evening – but this became increasingly difficult. The first casualty was meditation; I did not have the energy anymore.

It is difficult to describe the mental lethargy known as chemo brain; at its worst, I experienced it as a total mental exhaustion – almost as if I no longer existed, having been finally reduced to the operator of a complicated and ungovernable piece of machinery inside which I was trapped. Fortunately, this extreme did not usually last more than a couple of days, about three days after the latest infusion. At its mildest it was a kind of light-headed, forgetful state of disconnectedness.

The second casualty was my usual level of physical activity. At the beginning of chemo, I managed 800 metres in the pool most days, but that was far short of the 1800 to which I was accustomed. Eventually, I had to stop swimming as the chemo exacerbated my recurrent chlorine intolerance.

Worst of all was walking. Docetaxel is infamous for inducing severe fatigue in the legs, so that sometimes I could not walk more than a few hundred metres in a day. One day I found myself stranded halfway between Victoria Park and the LBC (approximately 500 metres). My legs would not move and I was forced to rest repeatedly so that I could progress by short stages. It took me so long that I was seriously concerned that I might not make it back.

A few days later, having walked just a few hundred metres for my first appointment, I told my acupuncturist that I might have to get a taxi back.

'Don't be absurd; of course, you will walk back' is not what Niccala said, but it's what the sparkle in her eye accompanying her actual words communicated. And I did walk back – with a spring in my step, but with a warning that it would only be a temporary fix. Still, as far as I was concerned she had performed a miracle. My twice-weekly sessions with her, or occasionally her colleague Jessica, were a blessing that greatly helped to relieve the more severe chemo side effects and buoy up my energy.

Being hampered by my legs shifted my perspective on life yet again. I could only walk very slowly, and it took several attempts during the first few weeks to get the pace right. But it was not just me that slowed down; the world slowed down with me. I saw things as an enfeebled old man; familiar things took on a different hue; once more I was seeing the world afresh.

Rotting

One morning I gave a slight tug at my hair and a handful came out. It was still clinging to my scalp by its rotting roots, but only just. I tried a second and a third time and more came off. It was clear that if I continued my head would be painlessly stripped bare within hours, and so I called in my barber, Luke, who clipped it all off in a few minutes. (With unwarranted zest, I thought.)

'You look so much better, Devamitra! It really suits you.'

'Huh', I snorted, unappreciatively – all the more so as I later discovered that he seemed to have triggered a reprise that spread rapidly around the LBC.

Two and a half years of continuous growth was then gathered and dumped in our bathroom bin, where it sat on top of the other detritus like an abandoned wig. And I walked away, a born-again skinhead, my elf-like ears, shorn of their cover, making me look more mischievous than ever.

If only my nails had come off so easily. First to go was my right thumbnail after I had caught it on a piece of cardboard. But it only partially lifted off, which made it much worse, causing me further discomfort. As I looked at the rest of my nails, it was clear that they were all going to come off eventually. It was the natural consequence of the neuropathy affecting my fingers and toes; my fingertips were too tender to fasten buttons or press the keys of digital locks painlessly.

Watching my nails slowly rot was a kind of contemplation of decay and regeneration, a metaphor for death and rebirth. It put me in mind of the traditional Buddhist meditation on the ten stages of the decomposition of a corpse. This is just one of many practices in which one reflects on death – strong medicine and definitely not recommended for beginners! Constant reflection on death and impermanence can aid the development of a more detached attitude to the body, which, ultimately, we have to surrender, but one needs to be in an emotionally positive frame of mind, otherwise it may be counterproductive. Instead of rising to the sublime state of equanimity, one may plunge into depression. But here was I, almost forced by circumstance to observe the process of decay affecting a live body – mine.

To persevere through so many minor trials, while simultaneously retaining a positive outlook, requires a lot of support that many people lack, but I was very fortunate. My community members gave me all the help I needed without reserve – not just free haircuts. I was relieved of all chores, and if there was anything I needed it was promptly provided. I was even chided for doing things for myself that others were only too happy to do for me.

I have never received such continuous kindness in my life – not just from my community, but from many associated with the LBC. Whatever rigours I might have faced, they certainly helped me to maintain my generally buoyant mood and I was truly grateful for all the cards, messages, flowers, and small gifts I received.

Second infusion

When I arrived at the hospital for my second infusion with Muditasri (an old friend originally from St Kitts in the Caribbean), a young Spanish nurse took charge of me and cannulated me. Shortly afterwards, Teddy arrived in a sorry state. He'd been up all night with diarrhoea. As he was rather stout and elderly, the nurse helped him on to his chair and then had the unenviable task of telling him that his medication would be delayed by an hour. It was more than the poor man could bear and he exploded.

She did her best to calm him down, but he had got himself into a foul mood. I quietly watched the whole scene. Finally, she freed herself from him and came over to check my drip. I whispered, 'Well done; such kindness, such patience! … I have the greatest admiration for your profession.' She squeezed my arm in silent appreciation.

I was sorry that she had been subjected to this unnecessary outburst, but so was Teddy, once he had had time to reflect, and he apologized profusely. Throughout the whole of my treatment I never saw any of the nurses lose their patience with any of their patients.

Muditasri and I left the hospital at lunchtime, which left me with plenty of time to consider what I might say to the Dharma-night class at the LBC that evening. The talk I gave proved to be perhaps the most popular I have given since my return to London in 2015 after many years based in Birmingham.

Ollie Brock (a few months later ordained as Prajnamanas) and Maitreyabandhu had come with me to the hospital for my first round of chemo. Muditasri accompanied me not only for the second but also for the third. Thereafter I preferred to go alone, as there really was no objective need for anyone to be with me. This is no reflection on my friends, or on their kindness and concern (which was deeply appreciated), but somehow I was able to relax more in the anonymity of the ward.

Perhaps this is why the idea of dying alone in a remote place has such a strong appeal for me. Should I ever feel death calling (I mean within a matter of days or hours, not months or weeks), then I suspect solitude would enable me to ease more into it and, assuming I was not bedridden or incapacitated in some other way, I would probably seek it.

Solitude has been such an important aspect of my life – like an old friend from childhood. I have done many solitary retreats of never less than one month's duration, the longest being nine months. Perhaps the circumstances of my early life had predisposed me towards seclusion. I was raised without siblings, and my school career protracted itself through eight different schools. As a result, I lost my new friends almost as soon as I had made them, which, in time, rendered me an inadvertent outsider and left me extensively alone.

*

Although I had not been told, the second dose of docetaxel was considerably higher than the first – a jump from 108 to 148 milligrams. The initial lower dose was precautionary, just in case there were any adverse reactions, but thereafter I received the full dose, which was calculated according to my body weight. This sharp increase caught me unawares, and it was then that I found it difficult to walk as my fatigue level took a quantum leap. Suddenly my body felt very old and I shuffled along streets and corridors like a nonagenarian, as if I had been given a preview of old age. This extreme phase only lasted for three or four days during each cycle, but it was seriously debilitating and a great test of my patience. I could go nowhere; I was housebound.

I spent endless hours lying down alone in my room, drifting in and out of a doze, occasionally reflecting. Even when I was brighter, I often lacked the concentration to read or to write due to chemo brain and frequently eased my mind by listening to music. The Romantics, principally Beethoven, Liszt, and especially Schubert, matched my mood of the moment.

One of the great ironies of chemotherapy is that, although it is a treatment, I experienced it more as a chronic illness. Thus far, the disease afflicting me, serious though it was, had barely troubled me. It had caused me no direct pain or discomfort, although in due time without treatment it would do so before finally killing me. Yet the treatment itself reduced me to an invalid.

All my life I had been blessed with health and vigour, yet I had been enfeebled so quickly, so easily. I was beginning to appreciate what Siddhartha (the young prince who became the Buddha) had seen when he encountered old age, sickness, and death, seemingly for the first time. True, I am still alive, but death has felt intimately close.

One morning I woke up feeling uncharacteristically grouchy as my mind wandered in and out of petty grievances. They were so petty I am embarrassed to recount them. This dragged on for over an hour until I caught myself. What was going on? Such thoughts had become alien to me; why had they returned unbidden? There must be some deeper significance, as indeed there was. For three weeks, I had not had the strength to walk to Victoria Park and I missed it badly, missed the contact with nature. I had to get there somehow for the sake of my mental and spiritual health, and I determined to do so.

I had been warned by a chemotherapy nurse that I must not try and push through the fatigue in the way an athlete might when training or competing, because this was of a different order. I decided, therefore, to walk to the park in short stages, no matter how long it took, resting whenever my legs felt as if they were about to seize up.

When I finally reached the park, my spirits soared as a surge of energy carried me forward, amongst the Sunday crowd, into the warmth of the sun, down the avenue of trees, beneath their shade, across to the pagoda, along the wooden bridge to gaze into the lake and laugh at the quarrelling coots.

The consultant and her registrar

Every three weeks, I met with the consultant, or her registrar, to be cleared for the next infusion, which would follow shortly afterwards.

'To my embarrassment, we have not met before', the consultant said as she greeted me with a warm smile a few days before my second round, 'but I know a lot about you.'

'Then you have the advantage over me', I responded jovially.

'Let me introduce you to my new registrar', she continued. It was only then that I noticed the silently attentive *devi* sitting beside her. Obviously of subcontinental extraction, though in most respects she seemed thoroughly English, she had the natural charm common to many Indian women. I sensed that some of my future consultations would be with her and I knew at once that we would get on well.

Among other things, I was expected to consult them about supplements. The general advice was not to take any. However, Niccala, my acupuncturist, had been encouraging me to take several. Chemo was my priority and I was unwilling to compromise that in any way, but I was happy to run her suggestions past the consultant.

'A few whacky questions for you', I said.

'Fire away.'

'Frankincense oil rubbed into the roof of the mouth.'

She laughed. 'Why?'

'Supposed to destroy cancer cells.'

'There's no scientific evidence', she insisted. (Niccala asserts that there is plenty. *I* know nothing, but I'm game for anything – even broccoli sprouts.) 'It won't harm you, but it won't do any good. I can't imagine what it would taste like.' And she clearly had no desire to find out. 'It won't get into the blood stream, you know.'

'Tincture of wild lettuce?' She looked puzzled. 'To calm restless legs', I explained, feeling myself on firmer ground. She shrugged.

'Magnesium oil for the same purpose.'

'Well, yes. I have heard that does work.'

We then moved on to the routine business as she asked whether I had had any nausea, vomiting, breathlessness, neuropathy, and I forget what else.

*

When we met again, three weeks later, although I was only halfway through the chemo, it was now necessary to start organizing the radiotherapy. The consultant explained that the intention was to give me the maximum dose of thirty-nine sessions spread over almost eight weeks. Finally, she said encouragingly, 'You are dealing excellently with the chemo.'

But, however well I might be coping with it, something was wrong – not with my body, but with my mind. I knew and recognized the problem, but did not know how to fix it.

3

Chemo *Sostenuto*

Several years ago, Punya was diagnosed with terminal cancer. I believe he was given eighteen months to live, but before he died he wanted to return to England to say goodbye to all his old friends, me included. When we met, I felt immediately that something had changed. He was animated by an urgency that I had never seen in him before; all that mattered to him now was the Dharma.

Eighteen months later he was still alive when I travelled to Boston to interview a Vietnamese Buddhist monk, for a book I had hoped to write. Punya met me at Logan Airport and drove me to his home. The moment we met I sensed that there had been another change, but I said nothing. I just watched him as he drove along. Finally, I broke the silence, 'What happened?'

He laughed. 'I could see it was on your mind.' He shrugged, sighed, and simply said, 'You adjust; become habituated. You forget.' Seven months later he was dead, but, before he died, he had remembered again.

I did not want to adjust and forget, but I sensed it happening. All the signs were there; I had forgotten the cancer, and my mind had become preoccupied with trivia. Certainly, the ulcerated skin on the most delicate part of my male anatomy was unpleasant, but it was hardly life-threatening. The large hardened swelling just below my navel was indeed tender, but was localized and clearly a reaction to my latest leuprorelin injection. Yes, the scarlet vein on my wrist was unsightly, but it was not even painful, so why the anxiety? (It had been damaged by a tiny amount of chemo leaking at the beginning of an infusion, I later learned from my consultant.) If I was to get anxious about anything, should it not be the cancer? Admittedly I checked the anxiety as soon as I was aware of it, never allowing it to take me over, but I did not know how to counter the underlying complacency of which I deemed it to be symptomatic.

Perhaps I expected too much of myself. The period and process of diagnosis had induced a state of heightened awareness that I had endeavoured to capitalize on, but it was difficult to sustain over an extended period. It's analogous to bereavement. The immediate pain of grief fades with time and is eventually forgotten. I knew I had lost the edge that had driven me dramatically forward. Constant reflection no longer seemed to bite in the same way, but then occasionally something would briefly jolt me back to reality, as happened on my fourth session on the chemo ward.

Fourth infusion

When I arrived, I was taken straight to a treatment room as I had one of the first appointments. I was then told that there would be a delay as the computer system was down for the fourth successive day. However, the nurses wanted to get everything in place so that, if the system revived, they could move things along swiftly. It was 9.30am and a cannula was once more inserted into one of my veins, where it remained for many hours as computers remained unresponsive.

By early afternoon the nurses were getting restless. They had had nothing to do all day, and nobody knew whether any of us would be treated. Later patients were being sent home; among them were many unhappy people, some of whom had become angry with the staff.

I had no more reading material, having slowly worked my way once more through Shakespeare's *Winter's Tale*. I had seen Declan Donnellan's production of the play a few nights before and had been irritated by his imposition of fashionable ideology on the text. Perhaps these ruminations were precursory to what happened next.

I became anxious. Will I get my treatment? What will be the consequences if I don't? A succession of similar thoughts rumbled through my mind as I slowly paced up and down the corridor until I caught myself and felt ashamed. Samsara! Samsara!

'Samsara' is one of many Indian words that have infiltrated the English language, but what did it mean to me at that moment as a Buddhist suddenly trapped in such angst? Samsara is not merely the external world; it is also *me*. I had been confronted by my habitual, unthinking interaction with everything beyond myself, caught by life as we know it, with all its pain and imperfections – life that imprisoned me in my unconscious response to a perceived threat to my well-being. I had been trapped yet again by everything that has moulded and conditioned me since time immemorial – by all that I strive to transcend. I had become abruptly locked into myself, held tightly in the constraints of self-concern that abides in the heart of every living thing, which hardens us to the needs of others and drives the worst excesses of humanity.

Samsara always goes wrong! This had been my mantra for decades, often saving my mental state in testing circumstances. Why had I forgotten it at the very time I most needed it? How foolish! I demanded of myself, 'What's so special about *you*? Why should *you* be treated ahead of others, perhaps at their expense? In the widest perspective, does it really matter whether you are treated at all?' … And then, remembering Santideva, a great eighth-century Indian Buddhist poet, scholar, and teacher, I reflected, 'Let others go before me, "I am medicine for the sick"…'⁴

I returned to the treatment room and sat on my chair as a deep tranquillity displaced the dark thoughts that had troubled me, leaving me perfectly happy to accept whatever the outcome might be. I wished the best for all – especially for the staff who were having to deal with a trying situation, not of their own making, sometimes without the sympathy and patience they deserved.

I chatted with the nurses who were frustrated because they could not help their patients. Because 'pharmacy' could not access computer records, 'pharmacy' would not release any medication in the absence of a handwritten prescription from the prescribing doctor. Those doctors who were present were all in clinic.

By mid-afternoon we knew that some of us would be given chemo, but we did not know who. It was not until 5pm that I was told that I was one of the lucky few and that my medication was being prepared. I was the second-last to be treated.

Just as I was about to leave the ward, the Filipino nurse who had treated me smiled and said, 'Thank you for being so calm.' I finally left the hospital ten hours after I had arrived, well past 7pm.

This incident had jolted my memory again; it had helped me to realign my emotional attitude, but it took something of great subtlety to reinvigorate my momentum.

Ida

The day before my third infusion, I had celebrated my sixty-ninth birthday, for which one of my young community members had given me a DVD of Pawel Pawlikowski's film *Ida*. Several weeks later we watched it together. It is one of the most beautiful films I have ever seen, and I can think of no other that has affected me so positively apart from Tarkovsky's *Stalker*. For weeks on end my mind had been preoccupied with old age (fatigue), sickness (chemo), and death. But *Ida* brought to mind Siddhartha's going forth in a surprising and uplifting way.

The film is set in Poland perhaps twenty years after the end of the Second World War. Anna/Ida is a novice Catholic nun whose Jewish origins are suddenly revealed to her by her last surviving relative. Her new-found identity precipitates a sequence of events that have a profound impact on her, but she meets each new challenge head-on and rises above them all.

For me, Ida embodied the spirit of going forth and I could see many parallels between the experience of the eponymous heroine and my own, enabling me to identify with her. I was reminded quite dramatically of my own higher purpose, which perhaps I had been in danger of forgetting. It is so easy to become self-preoccupied when you are confronted day after day by a succession of minor ailments such as those thrown up by chemotherapy. Although I had vigorously resisted any tendency in that direction, I needed *Ida*, at the time that I watched it, to stiffen my resolve. But the film did more than that; it renewed, perhaps deepened, my own inspiration.

Radio school

Tragedy and comedy are the stuff of life, and after the sublime tragedy of *Ida* I was next thrust into the comedy of a radiotherapy seminar, which certainly had its ridiculous moments. There were about twenty patients present, some with their partners. Everyone except me had undergone prostatectomy, and they would only receive four weeks of radiotherapy – half my dose. I was the only chemo patient.

A urology nurse introduced the seminar, which would explore four principal topics. First to speak was Rick, a young radiographer, who was later often on the team treating me. I took an immediate liking to him. He emphasized that we must all start training now as the bladder needed to be full at the time of treatment. 'It's no use coming if you can only hold 200 millilitres; that won't be enough and we won't be able to treat you.' The target was 350.

After Rick, the physio took over. The presence of women did not inhibit his slightly suggestive demonstration of how to identify our bladder muscles together with the exercises necessary to strengthen them. Discourses on the general importance of exercise and good diet followed, which I am sure would have been helpful to many of those present, but neither of which taught me anything I didn't already know.

I was beginning to yawn when at last we arrived at the entertainment: erectile dysfunction.

Apparently, James was to have been present to explain and demonstrate a vital piece of equipment but, unfortunately, he had not been able to come. The urology nurse looked distinctly uncomfortable as she explained this to us. As his stand-in, she was caught between a rock and a hard place, and my flagging interest was now suddenly aroused.

'Well… the important thing to remember is… use it or lose it, because… well, if you don't there is the danger of permanent loss of function… and it may shrink. After all it really is only a muscle and, like any muscle, lack of exercise will result in wastage.'

I could easily imagine the alarm hidden behind the impenetrable faces of many of the men present, some of whom, I suspect, were suffering from involuntary non-exercise of a possibly shrinking muscle.

Nurse continued at a rapid pace, perhaps in an attempt to get the ordeal over as swiftly as possible, 'Fortunately, we can help you... I mean, there are things we can give you. James should have been here to demonstrate how to use the pump... but we don't actually have a pump here at the moment so... well, if you do have any questions, do ask.' (Clearly, Nurse was not in a position to demonstrate anything. I wonder how James would have gone about it.)

There was an uneasy silence until one brave soul spoke up.

'I have a question.' Nurse smiled encouragingly, if somewhat uncertainly. 'I've tried the pump, but it didn't work.' Nurse was looking increasingly unsure of herself and, obviously at a loss for words, glanced desperately in the direction of her male colleagues. The physio gallantly sprang up.

'What happened?' he demanded firmly, yet sympathetically.

'Well, I read the instructions and... had a go, but it was really uncomfortable.'

'Ah, yes. You see, it's really important that you get a vacuum. It draws the blood into the, er... muscle. You just need to persist. Talk to me afterwards. Most men manage to get stimulated eventually. Any more questions?' No, just blank looks – except I had one for Nurse, which I was sure would be of no interest to anyone else and which I sincerely hoped would cause her no further embarrassment.

When the session had finished, I approached her and asked, 'Apart from shrinkage and loss of function, are there any other medical concerns about... not exercising?'

'Oh no, you don't have to', and then with an inquisitive look, 'but most men seem to want to.' I explained that I was a Buddhist and that for a period of twelve years, when I was much younger, I didn't. And there had been no shrinkage, I might have added, but perhaps that might have pushed my credibility a bit too far.

I approached the physio as I had an appointment with him.

'What's the problem?'

'I need help in managing fatigue.'

'That's unusual.'

'I thought it was very common.'

'Not really.' He quickly scrutinized me. 'How do you exercise?', he asked somewhat suspiciously, looking at me like a detective about to trap a criminal. I told the truth and he laughed. 'I see the problem. Most people don't even notice the fatigue because they don't exercise very much, if at all.'

Dancing the night away

Chemotherapy seems to exacerbate existing weaknesses and conditions. Restless legs syndrome (RLS), involuntary movement of the legs, was one of mine – especially at night when it can severely interrupt sleep. For me, RLS had previously tended to be mild and occasional; under chemo it became chronic and at times almost constant. I mentioned this to Niccala, and during one acupuncture session she concentrated specifically on treating it.

I was lying on the treatment table with needles in my legs and elsewhere, when suddenly my legs began to go and they would not stop. I looked down at them; although they were clearly not up for the cancan, they seemed to be attempting an Irish jig. I called out to Niccala, who was in an adjacent room, and she returned immediately and worked hard to calm them down.

'I've never seen anything like it', she said, with a hint of suppressed amusement in her expression; me neither – it was the worst it had ever been. 'Ask the oncologist if there's anything they can give you', she suggested.

*

'You need quinine sulphate', said the registrar the following day, 'but you are on so many drugs at the moment, I'm reluctant to prescribe any more. Try Indian tonic water.' Of course! I mentioned that my swimming coach used to recommend drinking it just before a training session to guard against cramp as it contains quinine.

'Oh, I used to love swimming', she said wistfully. I noticed the fitness tracker on her wrist and asked her about it. 'My husband bought it for me', she explained.

'What do you do for fitness now?'

'Nothing', she replied. 'I know I ought to.'

'Like so many of my medical friends… You would like to?'

'Oh yes, but it's so difficult getting started.'

'Just go to the pool!'

Radio consent

A few weeks later, the registrar began our consultation with a long preamble about radiotherapy, speaking rapidly, like an actor racing through lines to herself minutes before the curtain rises, as she explained likely side effects and post-treatment problems. This was necessary before I could sign the consent form.

'You realize that you will become infertile?'

'I'm almost seventy', I replied, wearily bracing myself for the erection question.

'Yes, but you see, I met with a man in his eighties a few months ago, omitted to tell him, and, when he found out later, he was deeply upset.'

'You're kidding!'

'Unfortunately not.'

'How absurd', I said, taking her smile as silent concord.

'… And you will also become impotent.' No surprise. Surreal, though, to hear these words in my seventieth year, enunciated in such a matter-of-fact way, by this beautiful young woman.

I gave my usual response, then signed away my genital prowess for this life without a twinge of regret.

And I can't be bothered with pumps. Such items may bring solace to a younger man, but, at my age, the very idea is ridiculous and prompts inner laughter that occasionally breaks the sound barrier into irrepressible mirth.

Cezanne to the rescue

A mere moment of inspiration can sustain you through the most difficult times. Often, such moments come unbidden, but you may also seek them out as I did shortly after signing that document seemingly so fatal to my manly pride. I had gone to the Courtauld Gallery, where I spent most of my time in a room in which a large painting by Manet hangs amid several by Cezanne. I absorbed myself in the Cezannes – the same paintings I had first enjoyed and learned to love fifty years earlier when I was a student, but now I saw them afresh.

I ignored the Manet until finally, stepping back to observe the whole wall, I could do so no longer. It is perhaps one of the best-known paintings in the collection, but its sensuous portrayal of a woman behind a bar at the Folies Bergère seemed so crude and out of place in Cezanne's company that I found it painful to look at.

Only then did I begin to see why some consider Cezanne to have been the greatest painter of modern times. His paintings seemed bursting with a hidden life that sprang off the wall into my mind and expanded consciousness. Perhaps only my current precarious state of health could have induced such heightened perception and gift me yet another precious moment.

Cyberattack

On the very day I consented to radiotherapy, just a few days before my fifth infusion, NHS services across the country were struck by a cyberattack. The hospital I attended was one of the most severely affected and so consequently, again, there was doubt about whether I would get my treatment on time. There were confusing messages in the media, and I received seemingly contradictory information from the hospital itself.

I was told not to take the steroid necessary before an infusion as I could be given it intravenously, should things work out, which they did. I had phoned the chemo ward on the day of my appointment and recognized the voice and accent of the Spanish nurse. She phoned back forty minutes later to confirm that I was on the list of the few to be treated and that I could go in at any time. However, there would be a delay of up to four hours as new blood tests would have to be taken and analyzed before we could be given our medication.

When I reached the treatment room, Teddy was already complaining about the delay on test results, which he could not comprehend. New tests were unnecessary in his case, anyway, he explained. 'Ask me ornitholigist', he demanded of the doctor who was trying to clear us all for treatment. 'She's seen me results and said they were okay.' But the 'ornitholigist' was not answering her phone. (Tweeting, perhaps?)

The doctor came over to me. 'Have you taken your steroids?'

'No', I replied. He frowned, but I explained why and later a Chinese nurse administered the usual rather high dose by the drip. However, I still had to take an additional half dose orally.

'You realize you won't sleep tonight', the nurse said. I laughed.

'I can't sleep even with the normal dose!'

Meanwhile, Teddy was getting increasingly restless and unreasonable. 'I can't wait four hours for them results. I've got an appointment this afternoon.' Several nurses, the ward sister included, explained to him that it was beyond their control, but the more they reasoned with him the angrier he became, insisting at frequent intervals that they should check for his results. After two and a half hours he got them and I was perhaps the unwitting beneficiary of his badgering as my results came through at the same time. At last he calmed down as a nurse administered his medication.

Again, he was ashamed, offered copious apologies, and then excused himself: 'I can't help it; it's me nature.' And once more the comedian emerged.

The nurse gave him his supplementary medication for the coming weeks. 'Do you need any anti-sickness pills?' she asked, offering him some.

'No, I don't get sickness. Keep 'em. Save the NHS 55 million quid.' She laughed, but then there was another problem. He was short, by two pills, of another medication that he really did need. At once he was anxious and immediately demanded the missing pills. Despite being told several times that they would be provided before he left the hospital, he insisted repeatedly that they get them immediately, working himself into a terrible passion as he did so. Consequently, he ended up with twice the amount of medication he needed.

This jolted him out of his madness, and once more he was overcome with remorse when he realized what he had done. Yet again he offered his excuse. 'I'm sorry, I just can't help it. I've always been like this. It's me nature.'

'I disagree', I said, from the opposite side of the room. 'You can change, but you've got to want to do so.' Suddenly everyone's eyes were on me. As he had just been released from his drip, he came over to me.

'How is that possible?', he asked.

'It's what I've been trying to do all my life', I replied.

'Oh yeah, I remember... You're a Muslim, aren't you?'

'Buddhist', I said, a smile escaping me; we then talked further as his mood softened.

'I greatly admire what you've done, but I made all the wrong choices in life', his last few words succinctly summarizing not just the tragedy of his own life, but that of human existence itself. Very few see, feel, or grope their way to the right choices; fewer still make them.

A few minutes later, after he had left, the nurses gathered together talking in subdued tones for the first time since Teddy's outburst had displaced the natural hubbub of the room with a wary silence. By this time, I had been discharged and so I went over to them. 'You do realize that you are much appreciated here, don't you?'

They smiled at my words, but then the Chinese nurse, who had had to bear the brunt of Teddy's anger, asked me, 'Why didn't you speak earlier?' Initially, I was taken aback and cannot recall whether or not I eventually did say what I certainly thought later.

Although she understandably found Teddy extremely difficult, I felt that she had dealt with his anger admirably well, but more importantly I had been waiting for the right moment to speak. I had not wanted to risk stirring his anger further by acting in a way that, in the heat of the moment, he might have perceived as interference and that in turn could have driven him to fury.

Secret blessing

When I returned home, Gus was in the kitchen. 'I got my fifth chemo!', I announced, delightedly, grateful to have been treated. He laughed.

'I can't think of anybody else who would be so pleased about that!' I could understand, yet I also wondered why. Although such thinking will be alien to many, Buddhist or not, is chemo not a secret blessing?

The overriding purpose of my life is to change for the better in the light of the Buddhist ideal of Enlightenment. But human beings rarely achieve new heights of humanity outside the context of suffering – which is just one reason why Buddhist tradition highlights life's harsher realities.

This is neither pessimism nor a denial of human happiness, but an acknowledgement that, however happy we might generally be, we cannot avoid unpleasant experience.

Suffering is the great challenge life throws in our faces, as if to say, 'deal with that!' In riposte, Buddhist tradition urges, 'Use it to your benefit; make the most of adversity!' Early in my Buddhist life I had learned that, if I could remain positive when facing life's difficult moments, this would transform my experience, making it easier to bear; more importantly, it would transform *me*.

When diagnosed with cancer, I had few options if I wished to survive. I could see no alternative to the treatments I had been prescribed; I certainly would have preferred not to be subjected to them, but I had made my choice, and it would be pointless to bemoan my fate. Even after four rounds of chemo, I had already been severely tried and tested, and my weaknesses had been exposed. As a consequence, my self-knowledge had deepened in a way that might not otherwise have been possible. Should I not therefore be pleased to have been given this opportunity and welcome it, as I try to do, with my customary enthusiasm and optimism?

Riding the fifth

The nurse had been right; I could not sleep that night. Dexamethasone had catapulted my mind into the stratosphere. I was in and out of bed for half the night until I could no longer be bothered to get back into it again. I did not feel a hint of tiredness until the following evening.

When my body and mind were finally reunited, I noticed something very strange. The horrible metallic taste that chemo leaves in your mouth had gone a stage further. I had completely lost my sense of taste, and my appetite had disappeared with it. It was with great difficulty that I motivated myself to eat, as it was such an unpleasant experience. Eating food that you cannot taste seemed a pointless exercise. Why would you eat if it gave you no pleasure? I had never realized just how much my sense of taste drove my appetite. My empty stomach was insufficient in itself to move me to eat. Fortunately, my loss was fleeting; after a couple of days my taste returned and I could eat happily once more.

However, a week later, things were seemingly taking a bigger downturn. The strength in my legs was not returning as I had come to expect, and other chemo side effects were much more pronounced and painful. Most alarming of all, I was beginning to weary of the whole process of chemotherapy. I had been immersed in it now for over three months. Was my spirit about to break, finally?

I confessed my weariness to a few friends, who considered this trough in my spirits perfectly understandable. Perhaps it was, but I was still dissatisfied with myself and became convinced that there must be some unacknowledged factor at work. Mulling it over, I realized that I had had no acupuncture for almost two weeks, as both Niccala and Jessica were away. Luckily, I had an appointment with Jessica the following day and she restored the energy to my legs.

Now I had no doubt just how much I owed to the dedication of my two most kind and generous acupuncturists.

*

Two weeks into my fifth cycle I was due to speak at the LBC's Dharma night, but the week before I had been plagued by chronic sleeplessness, caused by RLS, which, in turn, had been exacerbated by chemotherapy. I felt exhausted.

Just before I was due to speak, one of my friends looked at me concernedly and asked, 'Are you sure you can do this?'

'Of course. I just need to get started, but it won't be one of my best.' My topic was a famous incident from the *Vimalakirti Nirdesa*, a Buddhist text popular in China and Japan. Manjusri, an archetypal figure symbolic of transcendental wisdom, visits Vimalakirti, a lay follower of the Buddha renowned for his wisdom, and asks about his sickness.

How ironic; I had not chosen the topic, but, perhaps inevitably, I spent a good deal of time talking about my own illness, placing it firmly in a Dharmic context.

The talk was appreciated perhaps more for effort than for content. My theatre conditioning runs deep. I had been determined to speak, even if I had had to do so lying on a couch like Vimalakirti. The idea that 'the show must go on', regardless of personal circumstances, was still deeply embedded in theatre culture when I was working. Perhaps for this reason, I cannot recall ever having excused myself from giving a Dharma talk through ill health, though I have often stood in for others.

Cosmic joke

As chemotherapy proceeded, I found myself increasingly prone to laughter – the soft, chuckling variety, not the violent, belly-shaking kind – and I wondered why. Life seemed to be becoming more and more amusing. Why had I never noticed before that life itself is such a comedy? Why had it taken me so long to understand the huge cosmic joke in which we all participate?

I found myself laughing at small things: human foibles – both my own and those of others – and even those of animals. The squirrel at prayer while greedily munching its food could divert me as much as the gulls and geese battling for bits of bread cast into the lake in Victoria Park.

Perhaps inevitably, given my ill health, the absurdity and vanity of worldly endeavour struck me with greater force. My laughter was never tinged with contempt, but was often accompanied by poignancy. How sad that things should be the way they are, and that so often we fail to see beyond them. There is no comedy without tragedy.

Probably because of the cancer, I saw and felt the tragedy and comedy of my own life with increasing sharpness; the one reminds me of the seriousness of the human predicament, the other lightens its burden; unified in their transcendent beauty, they can give rise to wisdom and compassion when keenly observed.

*

I was due for an MRI scan later on the same day that I met with the registrar for the routine consultation a few days before my final infusion. 'Presumably the scan will show whether or not the chemo has shrunk my tumour.'

'Oh, it will have done something! Otherwise, why put yourself through all *that*?' Indeed. The scan would enable the radiotherapy to be precisely targeted.

There was nothing else to discuss and so, as we had several minutes to spare, I advised her how to establish a regular exercise routine, warning that I would be quizzing her as to whether or not she had succeeded when next we met.

'Good. That will give me an extra incentive to actually do something.'

'Perhaps involve your husband too', I added.

'Yes!' she responded seemingly delighted at the idea.

*

When I finally left the hospital, I could not help but wonder what my latest scan would reveal, as, despite my young friend's optimism, I was aware that chemotherapy does not always work. But it was pointless to speculate and I did not want such thoughts to distract me, so I put it out of my mind. I would find out in due course.

4

Chemo's Parting Kiss

'The third week of the cycle is your recovery week', a chemo nurse had explained to me in the early days of my treatment when I was still a chemo-innocent. 'We like to give you a short break so that your system can recover a little before you start the next round.' Pausing, she chuckled before continuing in a tone of mock cruelty, 'and then we hit you hard again!'

I was determined to take full advantage of these weeks when I had a bit more energy and could lead a more normal life. Just before my sixth infusion, making the most of my few days of freedom, I attended a concert featuring a late-Beethoven quartet and left with a lightness in my step that belied the fatigue still weighing heavily within my legs.

The following evening, I went back to the Old Red Lion Theatre in Islington, where I had performed the previous year. When I arrived, I was warmly greeted by Clive, the artistic director, who once again told me how positively he remembered my performance. I was not only flattered, I was deeply touched. Wondering how my performance might have left such a powerful impression on him prompted me to reflect.

The blood that had foreshadowed my cancer diagnosis had been flushed out with my urine while I had been rehearsing. It had haunted my mind then, its significance lurking on the periphery of consciousness like a watchful thief waiting for the right moment to abscond with my health or, better still, my life.

I had not then been willing to face the seriousness of its intent, and this must have influenced what was working out in rehearsal, eventually finding subtle expression in performance. There was an uncanny congruence in my immediate experience and that of the character I was playing, although I did not understand this at the time.

It's about porn addiction

Though I was often alone as I endured the chemo limbo, I also had many visitors, including several friends from beyond London, and I was greatly pleased to see every one of them. All of those meetings meant a lot to me, and I regarded them as vital elements in the extraordinarily supportive conditions that have borne me up and helped to carry me beyond the concerns of my ailing body.

Among my visitors were Debbie Korley and Vinta Morgan, my fellow cast members in *Further.Still*. I was truly moved that they had made the effort to come. Working together with Gus and two such seasoned actors had been a sheer pleasure to me after a break of forty-three years. Better still, again I had friends whose work I could go and see; that always makes theatre so much more enjoyable.

*

Debbie and I had had to work particularly closely together. As I never do things by halves, and because she is such a gifted and hard-working actress, we established a strong connection. She was currently rehearsing a play for the Blue Room at the Royal Festival Hall.

'I'll go and see it', I said.

'You won't like it', she warned.

'That won't stop me.'

'It's about porn addiction, Devamitra.'

'Pity… But that won't put me off!'

Sometimes they do get the results wrong

Two days after my evening at the Red Lion, I was back at the hospital. I had looked forward to 5 June as if it were my birthday. It was my last morning on the chemo ward – the beginning of the end of chemotherapy. However, as soon as I had sat down on the treatment chair, I was told that it may not be possible to treat me.

This time the culprit was not the computer system, or its hackers, but my own body. A test, taken a few days before, indicated that my white-blood-cell count was far too low. A new test would have to be taken and, unless there was a significant increase, they would have to send me home.

Shortly afterwards, Teddy arrived. Overcome by embarrassment, as he recalled his previous visit, he was apologizing to all the staff in sight.

'Don't worry, I'm in a good mood today, I promise yer. I won't give yer any problems.'

I glanced at him, then at the nurses. 'I'll make sure he doesn't', I said. Teddy laughed.

'Oh yeah. He won't give yer no problems, either. He's always very calm, he is.' Then he was put to the test. He too needed another blood test before they could proceed, but this time he was as good as his word and made no complaint.

*

Astonishingly, my white-cell count was now normal for the first time since I started chemo! Previously it had always been low, yet sufficient. The nurse seemed surprised by this latest result – and I certainly was.

And so I received my final infusion and left the ward for the last time a happy man, wishing well to the nurses and to Teddy. Sure, I had the final storm to ride, but that could not daunt me because I would not be going back for more.

But what could have so miraculously increased my white blood cells? The first test had been taken on the Thursday, but two days later I had acupuncture and I remember Niccala saying that she had wanted to prioritize boosting my immune system. Was this the explanation?

'Probably', she said when I saw her the following day, 'but, you know, sometimes they do get the results wrong', she continued rather modestly, her mild scepticism of Western medicine revealing itself momentarily from behind her wry smile.

Overpowering the rank refuse

The chemo ward was now behind me, but the chemo itself was not, and I would still be under its influence for four more weeks.

In the meantime, it was wreaking its usual havoc, especially inside my overburdened legs and my rotting nails, the latter tinged with an odious smell from the discarded tissue trapped beneath them. No matter how thoroughly I tried to clean them, their mildly faecal odour was as persistent as Lady Macbeth's damned spot. I could not rid myself of it, but… why should I try? Is it not the mark of death – with which we are all born and which cannot be washed away – made manifest? Was it not of benefit to me, this faint yet constant reminder not just of death, but of decay?

As the neuropathy afflicting my fingers intensified, attempting to pick up coins accidentally dropped to the floor became a major enterprise, invariably ending in failure, as my fingertips lacked grip. Best not to drop them in the first place, but this was not entirely a matter of unmindfulness; just getting hold of them properly inside my pocket required a skill that had deserted me and it could also be painful.

But worst of all, my restless legs were more hyperactive than ever – sometimes for hours without cease, especially at night. By 4am, if I was lucky, they would calm down and I could once more sink intermittently into delicious oblivion for an hour or two before it was time to rise.

Coping with insomnia is always difficult, but I am well practised; surrender is the only answer. But there are also perks.

One Sunday, rising at 5am, abandoning any further attempt at sleep, I went out onto the terrace adjacent to my room to get some fresh air. The morning chill enlivened my senses as I took in the surrounding scene. From behind a tower block, the sun was slowly revealing his splendour to a cloudless sky. Along a neighbouring roof, a solitary crow sauntered with not quite his usual swagger and sway, still caught perhaps in corvine dreams of corvine beauty. King of his television aerial, atop its highest point, a goldfinch released his ever-rising trill, proclaiming his faith to the Feathered Almighty on high – it was the Lord's Day, after all. Rising from the stillness below, overpowering the rank refuse nearby, the sweetest jessamine suffused the air and wafted me higher still.

*

Despite my sleeplessness and my errant brain, I was able to write most days, sometimes for several hours. My capacity for immediate response, so necessary for fluid conversation, was significantly retarded by chemo brain, my communication sometimes disjointed and somewhat haphazard. But writing is much more reflective. You can take all the time and space you require – two commodities I had in excess. Better still, at times my mind was uncommonly lucid, my perception sharper than ever.

Writing became a great solace to me, but it was also fun. Laughing at my predicament and my foibles unburdens me – especially if others laugh along with me, but, if it could *help* others, that would give it a value far transcending the diversion it brought me.

I am no more scared of cancer than I am of life

Several friends who had spoken or written to me had mentioned their 'cancer scares', prompting me to reflect on what this idea might imply. I had an instinctive aversion to it and needed to understand why.

A few years ago, on a long solitary retreat, I strained an intercostal muscle just above my heart. I understood that perfectly well, but my unconscious fears quickly attached themselves to the idea that I had a heart problem. They haunted me with increasing intensity for several weeks until finally I broke free of them. That was a heart scare, I suppose; but it had nothing to do with my heart.

When my blood had fled with my urine, I understood that it might have serious health implications and sought immediate medical advice, but, even when I was told that the blood could have come from a tumour, I did not have a 'cancer scare' – that would have obstructed or distorted my immediate experience.

Consequently, when I was finally diagnosed, cancer was not a 'scare' but the reality I faced. It did not scare me; I am no more scared of cancer than I am of life. It sobered me and concentrated my mind, enabling me to bring a Dharmic perspective to bear on it at once. Had I allowed it to scare me, I may have wanted to push it away, making it more difficult to face and ultimately more painful.

Thinking in terms of 'cancer scares' is just one symptom of the widespread, disproportionate fear of cancer that afflicts our society. If you have a 'cancer scare' you are not dealing with cancer, but engaging with an abstraction to which your unconscious fears have become attached.

When my father was dying of an enlarged heart, his cardiologist insisted that, in terms of health, people should most fear heart disease, not cancer. Much can be done to treat cancer, very little for heart failure.

But the tragedy of human life is much greater than cancer, or any other health issue. Our fears need a broader and deeper base. I do not fear cancer, but I am wary of falling into negative mental states: I fear my own potential reaction to cancer. That is far more serious than the cancer itself.

Know your enema

Before I could start radiotherapy, I had to go to the hospital for a dummy run so that, at my first session three weeks later, things could run to schedule. Shortly after arriving, I was greeted by Rick, the bright young radiographer from the seminar, who then took me into a consulting room and explained what was about to happen. But first he asked if I had any feedback on the seminar, as these events had only recently been introduced.

'Apart from your presentation, I learned nothing new, frankly', I said. 'I doubt I would have relished a demonstration of the erectile pump, had that happened', I continued, unable to hide my amusement at the idea, 'but I also wondered how the women present might have found it.'

'Well, there was a demonstration at the next one', he said. 'James was very good, he just came in and got on with it straight away, no messing.' He paused, unable to stifle his grin, 'Must admit, some of the women did look rather shocked when they left.'

And then down to business.

'Did you bring an enema?'

'Of course.'

'You'd be surprised how many don't.'

'I wouldn't! … But there's no mention of it in the letter.'

'Yeah. We need to fix that. Now, first thing we have to do is get you to evacuate your bowels. So, go to the toilet, use the enema, squeeze it all in and, if nothing happens after fifteen minutes, have a go anyway.'

'Right.'

'Then empty your bladder, go back to the waiting room and drink five cups of water in the cups provided so we know you've drunk the right amount. Okay? Then we'll call you through after twenty-five minutes and check your bladder.'

'We've come for radiotherapy'

I did as bidden, then sat down in the waiting room opposite a woman of my own age who was obviously very anxious about her husband, whom she had accompanied. I could imagine they had been together all their adult lives, but now their shared life was threatened by cancer.

'We've come for radiotherapy', she explained.

'Both of you?', I asked, slightly puzzled.

'No. Just him… We're already on immunotherapy.'

'I see.' I paused, not quite sure what to say next. 'Well, I hope it goes well.' She smiled at me rather sadly.

A little later, her husband returned and they left as wrapped up in one another as perhaps they had been all their lives. How would she cope without him, if he died? I doubted that she would have the resources to separate her own life from his. But I hoped I was wrong.

Eventually I was called by one of the radiographers. 'Devamitra?' I nodded, pleased she had got my name right. 'We're ready for you now.' But, unfortunately, I was not ready for them, as there was insufficient water in my bladder and so I had to return to the waiting room for a further twenty minutes.

This time, I found myself opposite a young woman who had obviously been observing me quite closely before she spoke. 'You a runner?', she asked, tentatively.

'No. Dodgy knees… Swimmer and cyclist.'

'I knew you did something.'

'How?'

'Well you carry so much sports equipment with you.'

'Do I?'

'Trainers, fitness tracker… But the real giveaway is the SIS water bottle.'

'Right!'

'And you're very trim.' I was flattered.

'You're a runner.'

'Yeah.'

'Here on your own?'

'Yeah. My husband is with the kids.'

'How many?'

'Two.'

She looked so fit, healthy, and full of life, but, like me, she must have cancer. 'I've just finished chemo', I volunteered.

'Me too. When?'

'Last week.'

'Then you're still in it.'

'Yeah.'

'How many rounds?'

'Six.'

'They gave me eight.'

'That's a lot.'

'Yeah.'

We lapsed into silence and smiled at each other.

She was then called by one of the radiographers and I was left alone to reflect. I had been strongly affected by our brief meeting and the potential tragedy haunting someone so young – and her family.

A few minutes later I was called again. This time my bladder was sufficiently full to proceed with the CT scan that was necessary to set up my treatment.

'Why didn't they offer you surgery?'

Several of my fellow Order members had been diagnosed with prostate cancer around the time of my own diagnosis, one of whom came to see me just as I was emerging from chemo. He had finished chemo a few months previously and his hair had grown back already; his nails, too. Naturally we compared notes and there was much that we had in common, but we spent relatively little time talking about chemo and the cancer it was targeting.

I was struck by the mutual shift in perspective that this life-threatening disease had effected. There is almost a sense of relief about it. You don't have to take life that seriously any more because suddenly everything is perceived as so much more precarious. Almost paradoxically, at least in my case, you can relax in a much deeper way, which is really quite wonderful, though difficult to sustain.

Everyone I knew who had had prostate cancer, unless it was at a very early stage, had undergone prostatectomy, but the procedure had not been offered to me and I never bothered to enquire why. But that did not stop my friends from asking *me*.

'Why didn't they offer you surgery?' asked one of my medical friends, incredulously.

I suppose it was a question I did not want to consider, but, in any case, I did not feel I needed an answer. When my friends suggested I ask my consultant, I thought that perhaps I should, but then I would forget about it.

Eventually, just as I was emerging from chemo, someone wrote to me who perhaps had a good reason for asking other than concern for my well-being and so I decided to respond, but all I could do was surmise – although of course, on a certain level, I had understood all along.

'Oh – I didn't realize that your tumour had spread beyond the prostate! Now I understand! Crossed fingers!!!' I appreciated the kindly, well-wishing sentiment, but crossed fingers? No. I don't want crossed fingers. Milarepa's frequent warnings against the terrible twins of hope and fear were ever present in my mind and I was determined not to fall prey to either.

The mirror's reflection and the pesky commuters

Before chemo people would always say that I looked much younger than my actual years, but, when I looked at my reflection in the mirror after the full course of chemo, a man significantly older than his actual years stared back. It was not just the absence of hair and the diminished eyebrows, there was a parchment-like quality to the facial skin; his eyes seemed more deeply sunken into their sockets; his ravaged face more in the grip of proliferating wrinkles, while the taut muscles surrounding his lips drew them slightly into the mouth, prophetic of the corpse to come. As I continued to gaze, Shakespeare's famous lines from Sonnet 73 came back to me:

> In me thou seest the glowing of such fire
> That on the ashes of his youth doth lie,
> As the death-bed whereon it must expire,
> Consum'd with that which it was nourish'd by.[5]

The moment I got back on my bike I was shocked. I had not cycled since just before my prostate biopsy seven months earlier, but now I could hardly pedal. Cycling a mere mile-and-a-half circuit exhausted me; swimming was equally draining. Yet a week later, I was cycling with ease, gliding through the rushing air beneath avenues of trees, in and out of the early morning sun, relishing the shifting warmth and cool caressing my bare arms and legs. Who cares if others could easily overtake me? Just give me a few more weeks and I'll show those pesky commuters.

Feeling energy thrill through my legs once more seemed a huge turning point. For more than four months, I had been legless – not from alcohol, but weighed down with chemo. I had dragged my reluctant limbs from place to place as if a hex had transformed them into marble stilts that might suddenly morph into a febrile tissue barely capable of keeping me upright, before shifting again into their ceaseless nocturnal frenzy. But now that my legs were slowly reviving and their restlessness diminishing, I felt particularly buoyant, even complacent; I was forgetting again. It was time for another reality check.

Another tumour?

My phone rang. It was a radiographer. There was an issue with my intestine, which was problematic for the radiotherapy. Consequently, my consultant had ordered a further scan and postponed my treatment. In the meantime, could I go to the hospital as soon as possible to collect a prescription? I was unable to go that afternoon, as I had an acupuncture appointment.

I did not quite understand the nature of the problem, even though it was explained to me – something to do with my small intestine being overfull. To me that suggested some kind of blockage. And immediately I was back on the edge – that uncomfortable place, so beneficial, yet so unappealing, where I must learn to stand fast.

'Have you found another tumour?' I asked the radiographer as soon as we sat down together the following morning. She laughed.

'Nothing so serious!'

'It was the first thing that popped into my mind.'

Such is the psychology of cancer, certainly as it affects me. Having one tumour, I am constantly alert to the possibility of more.

'No. The problem is that your intestine is very gaseous', she continued. (Could it be those accursed broccoli sprouts… or perhaps all the soya?) 'This means that we can't get it sufficiently clear of your prostate to give you the full treatment.' (But I *want* the full treatment.) 'If we did, the side effects would be very severe and, obviously, we don't want that.' (Hmm, I suppose not.) 'So, starting today, we want you to take a course of laxatives to try to dispel the gas.' (Good; let it be blasted to the end of the universe!)

'My acupuncturist has already done some work on my intestine', I added, immediately regretting it.

'Where were the needles inserted?' she asked, frowning. I told her. 'You must not have any needles anywhere near the pelvis, when you are being treated', she insisted.

'I'm sure my acupuncturist would not do that', I replied. Even so, she would need to check with my consultant about the acupuncture. Next, I was told the results of my recent MRI scan, as I had asked for them when speaking to her over the phone the previous day.

'The swelling has completely disappeared from the lymph nodes', she informed me, 'and the prostate lesion has shrunk significantly.' I felt hugely relieved (thus stepping back again from the edge, forgetting... How quickly it happens).

'So the chemo has done its job.'

'Yes', she smiled. 'It's a very good outcome.' How ironic: I had gone to the hospital braced for the worst, but would leave with mostly good news; better that way around than the other. Unfortunately, however, my consultant was insisting that there must be no acupuncture during radiotherapy, as 'acupuncture changes the way the body functions.'

A ghost, a bad omen, a man on the brink?

I was then given a prescription for the laxatives, which I took immediately to the hospital pharmacy and sat down to wait.

'Hello, Devamitra.' I turned to see someone I recognized from the LBC. 'What are you here for?'

I explained. 'And you?'

'I've just seen my consultant. My tumour's been downgraded from T2 to T1.' He looked greatly relieved.

'Good news.'

'What's yours?'

'T3b.' The expression on his face rapidly changed. His eyes seemed to retreat from me as if he was trying to get away. What lay behind them – fear, embarrassment, aversion, pity? What were they seeing – a ghost, a bad omen, a man on the brink? Having pushed me back on to the edge, he said goodbye.

Of course, I could have compensated with inner kudos getting all snottily, mentally uppity: 'T1! Call that a cancer?' Instead, as I waited for my medication, I recalled my own reaction, months before, to Jayamitra who had passed the point of no return from stage three to stage four. So far, I had remained on the right side of stage four, but I tried not to forget that others, despite treatment, had been at stage three only for some of their bad cells to migrate through their bones, or lymphatic system, and thrive elsewhere, with murderous intent, as stage four.

Eye of the needle

'But I've treated hundreds of people on radiotherapy; most find it really helps with fatigue. It's never been an issue', Jessica maintained when I told her the following day that the acupuncture had to stop. Clearly, I needed to speak directly with the consultant, but first I sought advice from two friends, both senior doctors. Although neither could speak authoritatively, they were not aware of any conflict with the treatments.

Several days later, just as I was about to be needled yet again, my consultant phoned. She relented about the acupuncture, but insisted that there must be no needles from my navel down to my mid-thighs, both front and back, during radiotherapy. It was to do with rounding up free radicals, apparently (a totalitarian purge, perhaps). This left me much happier, though no wiser.

She needed to see the result of my next scan before she could replan my treatment. Of particular concern were the lymph nodes, which needed to be hit hard, but that would not be possible if the gas persisted. The intestine must be well clear of the beam. This was normally achieved by a sufficiently full bladder pushing it out of the way, but the gas was preventing that.

It would be at least three more weeks before I could be placed at the mercy of that powerful radio beam. In the meantime, Jessica set to work – to blow the gas away.

'Phlegm!' she said.

'In my intestine?' I asked, doubtfully. She smiled inscrutably, her Chinese conditioning coming to the fore.

'Two kinds. Visible. Invisible.'

'This is invisible *phlegm*?' I asked, yet more sceptical.

'We can get rid of it.' As she rather charmingly put it, 'When your stools can pass through the eye of a needle, you will know it has gone.' Six days later, after I had consumed large quantities of organic vitamin C and 'Oxytech', the phlegm invisibly passed away.

*

Four weeks after my final infusion, I had celebrated my freedom from chemo with a talk to the LBC Dharma-night class on Vajrapani, an archetypal figure symbolic of spiritual power, or unbounded energy. There are many such figures in Buddhist tradition symbolizing different aspects of the Enlightened mind, and there are meditation practices associated with them all. All Order members in Triratna are initiated into one of these practices at the time of their ordination. Frequently visualizing these figures in meditation is a means of dwelling on the qualities they embody, thereby allowing them to influence you subtly and help you to develop them.

Vajrapani is most frequently represented in Buddhist art as a terrifying figure surrounded by fire. Such images can be shocking to anyone who thinks of Buddhism exclusively as a peace-loving tradition. It is indeed a non-violent teaching, but there is a destructive dimension to Buddhist practice that we cannot forget or ignore. The wrathful figures illustrate this and represent the destruction of everything that holds the individual back from spiritual progress: negative emotions, psychological conditionings, and ignorance. However, the violence that they represent is to be targeted by the individual at the contents of his or her own mind. To use such images to justify violence against others would be contrary to the spirit of Buddhism.

I relished the opportunity to explore this dangerous figure. I could have danced all night in Vajrapani's aureole of flames and savoured every moment. But how foolish of me to tempt fate so blatantly; Vajrapani cast his thunderbolt to rein in my intoxication. Though I had kissed goodbye to chemo, like a jealous lover, it would not let me go that easily and it gave me one last, nasty surprise – another lesion, this time much bigger, on that most delicate part of the male anatomy. It bled and it hurt. Huh! No more parting kisses for chemo.

5

Chemo's Ghost

Sariputta, one of the Buddha's two chief disciples, was once meditating in the open air on a full-moon night. A passing mischievous spirit, beguiled perhaps by the moon shining on Sariputta's freshly shaven head, found such a tempting pate irresistible and gave it a hefty swipe with his club. However, Sariputta was so deeply absorbed in meditation he felt nothing.

His friend Mogallana, who had seen the assault, asked him if he was in pain. After thinking about it, Sariputta admitted to a trifling pain in the head, but nothing more.

You may not believe in mischievous spirits, but I've seen them. They assume many forms, most frequently manifesting nowadays as fourteen-year-old boys on bikes.

A totally bald head was part of my immediate post-chemo legacy. One afternoon, while sitting on a park bench talking to an old friend, my naked head presented an easy and irresistible target for one such spirit as it passed swiftly by. Consequently, I received a hard slap on the back of my scalp, giving me a headache that was more than trifling. This malign spirit then took aim at another bald patch a hundred metres further on. As we all know, a real boy would never behave so badly, which is how I knew it was a spirit.

My hair's reluctance to grow was clearly a liability and my reviving beard was no protector, as beards are insufficient to frighten such wanton spirits, but, even if they could, my new growth was barely visible. And, anyway, I had started shaving again – not that there was much to remove; it was more an exercise in reassurance. Other chemo side effects also lingered – addled brain, leaden legs, neuropathy in fingers and feet – but all much milder than during treatment.

'You're going to Mercury, today'

The CT scan I had been given to determine whether or not my intestinal gas had been dispersed revealed that it mostly had, but there might now be an issue with my large intestine. Although there was still doubt as to whether or not I could have the full treatment, there would be no further delays. At the very least I would receive what had been the normal treatment a few years previously.

I started ten days later. 'You're going to Mercury, today' the receptionist told me, smiling sweetly at me as I checked in, having her little joke with a new patient. All the machines are named after planets, all equally powerful; Mercury is the latest model.

Once more the preparation routine was explained to me by a radiographer. 'Am I getting the full treatment?' I asked.

'You would not be here if you were not.'

'Good.'

Any doubt about treatment prompted mild, residual anxiety – it tripped me up every time – usually just a quick flash and then it was gone. It was like an alarm clock that awakened me, then I would remember that I had forgotten and had fallen victim again to complacency.

'Could I have a later appointment time? I need to fit in an early morning swim.'

'I wouldn't advise swimming. It could irritate the treatment area.'

A human water sprinkler?

My preparation completed, I reported back to reception, 'Ready for lift-off.' The older of the two receptionists looked at me quizzically, the younger, pretty one giggled.

Fifty minutes later, having put on a hospital gown, I was taken into the treatment room. My bladder was then checked to see if it was sufficiently full, which it was not. Twenty minutes later, having drunk two more cups of water, the necessary level was finally reached.

It took a few days to work out how much fluid I needed to be ready on time: three glasses of water first thing in the morning, followed by a large fruit smoothie mixed with muesli, a mug of decaffeinated coffee (caffeine was not recommended), another glass of water before leaving for the hospital then two more cups as soon as I arrived. After evacuating my bowels and emptying my bladder I then had to drink another litre of water as my immediate preparation.

Good job I was not about to have acupuncture – I might be at risk of becoming a human water sprinkler. But probably not; most of this fluid seemed to store itself in my body until night-time so that it could then slowly trickle into my bladder to keep me active half the night emptying it.

Anyone nicked it?

The door of the treatment room looked like it could resist a nuclear blast, it was so thick. Mercury itself was enormous and highly complex.

'Oh, it's just a load of plastic', Sangita, one of the two radiographers, pronounced, dispelling my awe.

'It'll circle you several times, with different parts moving in and out', explained Yasmin, her companion, 'but nothing will touch you.'

First they had to position me very precisely on the treatment table. To enable them to do this, I had been given three barely visible tattoos, during the dummy run ten days previously – one a few inches below my navel, the other two on top of each side of my hips. Two lines of intersecting green light projected down from the ceiling, forming a cross on my exposed pelvis, so that they could get the tattoos in alignment with the light.

My head, legs, and feet had to rest in moulds to ensure that I did not move. When they were satisfied, Sangita and Yasmin raised the table to what seemed to me to be their head height – they were both rather petite – then darted out of the room, always with the same parting words, 'Here we go!', just before that huge door closed behind them. Shortly afterwards the machine swung into action, circling me to take a scan.

After several minutes the position of the table was slightly adjusted from inside the control room to get my prostate in exactly the right place. A little later there was the sound of things clicking into position, followed by a sustained electronic buzz as the machine began to circle me again, this time delivering death and destruction to the cells it was targeting. Rotating through 360 degrees, starting and ending beneath me, it then revolved back in the opposite direction, completing the day's treatment. I was to undergo this procedure thirty-nine times – each revolution taking about forty seconds – a total of fifty-two minutes penetrated by the beam.

Mercury had cost the hospital one million pounds, excluding installation costs. 'They came one day to check that it hadn't been stolen', Yasmin claimed.

'Where did they think we would sell it', asked Sangita, her potential partner in crime. 'Ebay?' I don't think they were being ironic!

Cyril and the ladies

I didn't know Cyril's particular protocol, but he was always prancing around trying to empty something, bowels or bladder; I had too much delicacy to ask. Probably much older than his youthful looks – 'Black don't crack', says Muditasri – tall and heavily built, he cut a merry caper tiptoeing from Mercury, heading for the Ladies, opposite.

Obviously, he needed to empty something and the Gents was at the wrong end of the waiting area for a man in a hurry. His NHS gown swinging open at the back revealing his naked legs, he darted surreptitious glances this way and that, then grinned at me mischievously as he disappeared inside.

As Cyril emerged from Mercury on another occasion, having already taken advantage of the Ladies just a few minutes before, this time it was engaged; even worse, the waiting room was full. 'Get back in there!' bawled out a cockney voice.

'Do it in a bottle!' called out another amid the general mirth as Cyril headed for the Gents grinning all the way, utterly unabashed, gown swinging open, as usual, to reveal his black briefs. Cathy and the other ladies – with whom he was a great favourite – giggled with delight at the sight of his hind parts. Cyril was a man – no apology, no mistake.

Cathy, a bleached blonde, her face meticulously made up, was probably in her sixties, had an extremely girly voice, girly clothes, and a thick cockney accent. After Cyril's latest antics she left, as usual, for Venus.

I had seen no men go in there, just as I had not seen any women heading for Mercury – though, admittedly, I had seen them leaving Mars. 'Is Venus just for women?' I asked Yasmin. She laughed.

'No. They treat men in there as well, but most of our work is with breast cancer.' The Mercury team concentrate on prostate, bladder, and rectal cancer.

'Why is there no Pluto?'

'It was declassified; it's no longer a planet.'

'Really? … And Uranus?'

'Hardly appropriate', she said, grinning.

'Oh… I suppose not.'

A few days later, Cathy was chatting with a friend while Cyril sat aloof, as he often did, eyes closed, arms crossed, desperate to catch up on sleep.

('Eight times!' he had told me, 'eight times every night I get up.'

'I know what it's like', I had responded.)

'Come and join us, Cyril.' I could see his reluctance. Not the kind of man to enjoy conversation about babies and granddaughters, I suspect, but, graciously, he went over to sit with Cathy and her companion.

'Your inner geography is unstable'

I was on the table waiting for the beam to go around, but instead Sangita was back in the room. 'We weren't happy with our first scan', she explained. 'You were two millimetres out of position.' The machines are accurate to within half a millimetre. She and Yasmin adjusted me slightly. 'Can you hang on for a few more minutes?'

'Sure', I responded without thinking; not so easy – you must not move once you have been positioned. Sometimes, it seems an age before the beam finally hits you, and, for a man with restless legs that might commence a jig without notice, this was potentially problematic. Worse, I might fall asleep then awaken suddenly as my body jerks. Just to remain awake, I had to exert my will fully.

The following day, shortly after checking in for my fifth treatment, one of the senior radiographers came out to talk to me. I sensed a problem. 'Your bone structure has changed.' That sounded serious.

'Is that common?' I asked, sensing my bogey lurking in the background, keeping it at a distance.

'It happens. Are you still having acupuncture?' she asked rather suspiciously.

'Yes, but I cleared it with the consultant.'

'What for?'

'Fatigue.' She was obviously unhappy.

'Okay. We'll give you the treatment as normal today, but we'll have to get another CT scan to get a more accurate treatment map. At the moment, they are struggling to target you precisely.'

The radiotherapy department is alive with radiographers – seemingly dozens of them. Back in the scanning room another complained, 'Your inner geography is unstable.' (Like continental drift, perhaps? Different parts of my innards parting company?) 'Your large intestine is always full.'

'Well, I was told to have a "good breakfast" before treatment… Should I cut back?' She paused to consider.

'Don't change anything unless we tell you.'

Prurience

For over a month I had enjoyed a taste of the freedom to which I had been accustomed before chemo, but that was all about to change. The last weekend of this temporary release I went to see Debbie perform in *Prurience*. It was a piece of immersive theatre, with the actors dispersed among the audience, set up as a mock support group for porn addicts (the assumption being that everyone present was an addict).

The rather camp 'facilitator' invited us all to participate and then proceeded to conduct the meeting in the 'New Age' style of many such groups. It was an extremely funny piece of satire, which triggered my sense of humour uncontrollably.

Many people seemed unsure – should anyone be laughing at this rather sensitive issue? I had no choice, having a politically incorrect sense of humour. The more I tried to stifle my laughter, the louder it would explode and, according to Gus, who had come with me, it persisted for about five minutes, sparking several others including him.

But it's uncomfortable if you are seemingly the only one laughing. It had happened to me once before, decades ago, at the premiere of Edward Bond's play *Lear*, but, on that occasion, I had been alone and several people had scowled or tut-tutted at me for the disturbance. They were oblivious to Bond's obvious irony and I delight in irony, as I do in satire, both in theatre and in life, unfashionable though they have become.

Debbie had recognized my laugh at once. 'It was great!' she said afterwards. 'It helped warm up the audience.' I had not laughed so much for a long time.

Chemotherapy? Had it. Radiotherapy? In process. Porn therapy? Don't need it. Laughter therapy? Can't get enough.

Four plus five equals hospice

The following morning, I caught an early morning train to Colwall to see Bhante at Adhisthana, the retreat centre in Herefordshire where he lived. Had I not taken this opportunity, I would have had to wait perhaps several months before I would be able to go. I was so pleased to see him again.

We discussed his recent writing, then I mentioned my memoir of the early days of Triratna.

'Well I hope you tell it as it was', he said quite firmly. Naturally, I shall do my best. I would not wish to do otherwise.

*

A retreat had just started the evening before and, on seeing me, an old friend approached and asked how I was getting on. 'You know, *I* had prostate cancer', he said. 'What's your Gleason score?' (The Gleason scale is a gradation of prostate cancers from mild to aggressive.)

I did not like talking about it; I never do – but I could hardly not answer.

'Four plus five', I replied.

'Same as me… And I'm still here', he said, smiling at me as living proof.

(Yes. And so am I… but it's early days. And anyway, what does it matter if I am not 'still here' in a few years' time? It will not be that much longer before I am gone, whatever happens.)

Once more a flash of anxiety had jolted me. My friend's words were meant kindly – perhaps as reassurance or encouragement, but I neither seek nor want either.

'If you ever need to talk about prostate cancer, just give me a call.'

(Yes, of course… but I knew I would not. Why? Why do I dislike talking about it? Do I still feel too close to the edge for comfort? Edge of what… existence? And what has comfort got to do with anything?)

'You know what they say about "four plus five"?' I didn't. He told me. All I recall was the word 'hospice'. And that was enough. I had remembered again and I was grateful for that.

The ghost

I cycled to the hospital every day during the first couple of weeks of radiotherapy. The last day I did so, Cyril noticed me heading into Mercury with my cycling gear.

'You didn't cycle in, did you?'

'Sure.'

'How did you manage that?'

I paused pensively then replied with a smile, 'I've got legs.' As I disappeared, the waiting room erupted with laughter.

'What are you laughing about?' Yasmin asked as I entered the treatment room.

Unfortunately, the following day, the fatigue in my legs, which had so plagued me during chemo, had returned with a vengeance and my few weeks of freedom were at an end. Once more I could no longer walk to Victoria Park.

Your enema is your best friend

Having to use an enema every day could be hazardous (especially if you have a haemorrhoid; I spare you the details). After three weeks, the effects were lingering well into the afternoon so that I dared not be too far from a loo.

'What are you eating?' Sangita asked. I told her. 'Cut back on the fruit', she recommended before taking me through to Saturn – I was temporarily switching planets; Mercury had swung out of orbit.

'Nice to see a different part of the universe.'

'Oh, it's just a slightly older model', she replied. It was slower, noisier, and less sleek.

Me playing dead all the while, this great, lumbering electromechanical beast cranked into place for the scan, groaning as it extended its arms before circling me, penetrating my innards with its eye, not liking what it saw.

The treatment table jerked forward then lowered as Sangita returned. 'Your bowel's too full', she complained, slightly sternly. Further evacuation was necessary. I scampered off to the loo, Cyril-style. The beast had a second look. It was just empty enough.

'What do you have for breakfast?' Sangita asked after the treatment.

'Mostly fruit.'

'Eat lots of stodge instead.' The following day, before my only trip to Jupiter, I did. 'Perfect!', Sangita cooed.

A farce of my own making?

One problem solved, three more to confront – that's the way with cancer treatment. The fatigue in my legs seemed to be slowly getting worse and, coincidentally, my GP had called me to the surgery to discuss blood-test results taken for my annual hypertension review.

'You're mildly anaemic', she told me. 'We may need to put you on one or two supplements.' And, of course, my blood pressure had gone up, probably as a result of chemo. 'The anaemia could be a factor in your fatigue', she added.

I phoned a radiotherapy nurse. 'What's your haemoglobin count?' she asked.

'118.'

'That won't cause fatigue.'

'Could it be the radiotherapy?'

'Not fatigue like that. I've never encountered it. It's probably lingering chemo.'

'But it eased off during the break between chemo and radio.' Now she seemed uncertain.

'Ask to see one of the doctors when you come in next.'

I called a chemo nurse. 'Chemo stays in your system for about six months', she said.

'But why would it ease off and then return?'

'Well look, if it gets any worse over the weekend, go and get checked out at your local A&E.'

A few minutes later she called back, 'I think you should go straight to A&E.'

'But why?'

'It might be something spinal. Best just check it out, for your own peace of mind and mine.' I now recognized her voice. She had sent me off to A&E unnecessarily before.

Dayanatha, a young doctor who lives in the community above mine, kindly came downstairs and examined me. 'No. Nothing spinal.' Good. I could forget about A&E. But the chemo nurse could not.

'Did you go to A&E?' she asked later that evening.

Was this farce of my own making? I could not help but wonder. It was so reminiscent of what had happened when I began chemo.

I simply wanted to understand what was going on, I had told myself. But actually, that was a tired old rationalization I had used too many times in the past, masking my profound unwillingness to face the uncertainty of existence. Too frequently, it seemed, I would do anything to distance myself from it, preferring to wallow in the cowardly comfort of complacency. But that was unworthy of my higher aspiration.

No magic solution

The fatigue worsened over the weekend. As I was not quite halfway through radiotherapy, I could easily imagine that, like a friend's sister, I might not be able to walk by the end of it.

Of all the side effects I had endured through cancer treatment, this was the most alarming. The fatigue I had experienced with each chemo cycle always began to recede after a few days, but this was worsening by the day.

When I reached the hospital on Monday, I felt very weak, mildly nauseous, and dizzy. One of the nurses examined me then consulted with a doctor. I should not be experiencing this level of fatigue, I was told. Unfortunately, my consultant was at another hospital and so I had to wait another two days before I could see her.

'The haemoglobin level is not a problem', she insisted. 'Chemo hits the bone marrow extremely hard. It will slowly recover without the need for any supplements', she continued. 'As for the fatigue, your body has been hit with one severe treatment and now you're receiving another. That's the problem.'

At last, someone at the hospital understood. This was exactly what Niccala had said to me when giving me acupuncture the day before.

'There's no magic solution.'

'So I just have to ride it.'

'Yes… And rest up!'

*

I did not relish the prospect of being unable to walk, but, my enemy now having been clearly identified, I knew how to fight it and I carefully chose my weapon. I hired a wheelchair later that evening from Wheelfweedom. (Profuse and most heartfelt apologies to the company for such an unforgivable spelling mistake. I hope they won't sue me.)

But I was still struggling and could not understand why, until I realized that I needed to speak frankly with my community. I would have to rely much more heavily on their help than before. I would need them all to do a lot for me, perhaps even help me up the stairs; I had already given up trying to climb them and was now going up backwards, pushing myself up each stair using my arms.

As I expected, they responded magnificently. A burden was lifted from my mind, and my characteristic buoyancy reasserted itself. I had suffered the worst dip in my spirits since my cancer saga had begun, and I needed to make more effort to ensure it did not happen a second time. I had allowed my mind to dwell on the possibility of life without the use of my legs. Again, I had been distracted from the cancer and the deeper, threatening issue beneath it – my own impermanence. I had lost yet another battle in the raging war between Reality and my intractable self-clinging.

Self-clinging

Self-clinging is the deeply ingrained belief in a permanent, unchanging self, often called a soul in religious contexts, but which does not exist according to Buddhist analysis. Just as our bodies gradually grow old even to the extent that it can be difficult to identify the young man of twenty-two with his later incarnation as a seventy-two-year-old, it is perhaps even more difficult to identify the common elements in their mental landscapes, even though we know there has been a continuity. If we give close attention to our mental states, especially when meditating, it is easy to see that there is nothing that is constant within them; they are shifting and changing all the time. Even during the course of an hour, but certainly throughout a day, we may experience happiness, contentment, restlessness, resentment, and a whole range of sentiments and moods in between. Perceptions are equally inconstant, and memory comes and goes like a ghost, assuming different guises as time passes.

Like everything else in the universe, all these things are subject to the law of impermanence; ultimately, therefore, there is nothing in our experience that we can claim to be 'me'. But that does not stop us from doing so and from identifying with our immediate experience, asserting it as 'mine'. We do not do this consciously; it is our habitual way of being – it is automatic, mechanical, and blind. And to see this pattern just for a moment can be terrifying; it undermines the deepest sense of security we have and threatens the stability we crave. This false sense of permanent selfhood, driven by the self-clinging that underlies it, is the source of all manifestations of human selfishness and all human conflict, whether between nations or between individuals.

Consequently, when I realized that I had once more fallen victim to self-clinging, it was salutary. It was a battle I had lost countless times and one I shall lose again and again, but I value those rare moments when I can see with growing clarity the source of all my own suffering. With increasing awareness, one day I may finally see through it and be free of its terrible grip.

Beauty is where you find it

'What an uninspiring view', a visiting friend had said months before as he looked out of the window of my room. Accustomed to gazing at the hills and sheep surrounding his isolated home, perhaps all he saw was a block of flats, terraced houses, and the forbidding facade of an old school building enclosing the view.

But now, recalling his comment while lying on my back and looking through that same window, I could see nothing but infinite blue sky, white clouds drifting across.

I sat up and looked again. The outlook was far from beautiful, but I had gazed at it for countless hours and had found beauty within it nonetheless – and beauty is always a source of inspiration to me; many times, it had touched me – especially when housebound and I had nothing else to look at.

*

I saw three trees; I've watched them morning, noon, and evening – in twilight, in sunlight, in shadow. I've watched their bare branches spring to life, sporting the tenderest green, brightening into the brilliant hues of summer, softening to the muted tones presaging autumn, clusters of seeming-orange keys – of the tallest, grandest of the three – darkening its leaves further. I've watched all three sway with the wind, whether in wild protest or gentle surrender; I've seen them battered by the rain.

Crows and magpies perched on chimneys, or squabbling along rooftops; pigeons seeking shelter in the foliage, gulls or swifts soaring high above, parakeets darting by; goldfinches and blackbirds searching for food; a lone heron lumbering through the air; a squirrel squatting on a rail, cheekily observing me; I've seen them all through that window and more besides. They have inspired me with the thrill of life.

I might not have been able to walk, but I did have a wheelchair and friends to take me for a spin. Even better, I didn't need to look where I was going and was free to let my eyes seek the hidden beauty that surrounded me when trundling along the avenue of trees leading to the park.

Where the planes completely overarched the road, I gazed upwards and felt dwarfed by their grandeur, astonished by their elegance; never before had the mottled beauty of their peeling bark seemed so vivid.

'With this, you don't even know if you'll be here next week'

I could no longer travel by bus for my treatment as I lacked the strength to walk the short distance to and from the bus stops, and I was now dependent on hospital transport. Sometimes that would be a car, at others an ambulance – an excellent service where I met and got to know other patients and some of the drivers.

I was often struck by the sanguine attitude of terminally ill patients. Jean, for example, probably about my age and formerly an actress, was so bright and genuinely cheerful, despite her evident pain. She had had a large tumour removed recently from her thigh, making it very painful for her to walk.

'When you get something like this [metastatic lung cancer] it shifts your perspective on life.' She clearly meant for the better, as her ready smile demonstrated. The last time I saw her shrunken form, she wished me well; then, 'Maybe we'll meet again', she said, 'but with this, you don't even know if you'll be here next week.' I'll never forget those words, nor the sweetness of their accompanying smile.

Some, unfortunately, bore their burden bitterly, or fell victim to depression, but many, perhaps most, were optimistic, and there was an abundance of mutual well-wishing, as one often finds between those facing a common misfortune.

Although I would never wish it on anyone, facing a life-threatening disease, like cancer, had a noticeable humanizing impact on many of its victims, perhaps bringing the best out of them, highlighting their fortitude and other strengths they themselves might never have suspected they held in reserve.

Dread-legs

Within an hour after each radiotherapy session, my legs felt as if most of the life had been blasted out of them. Taking the few steps to the toilet was exhausting – but at least I could do that.

The chemo had mostly affected my thigh muscles, but the radiotherapy had penetrated down to my calves, the sensation more severe, filling them with dread at the prospect of moving; it felt as if iron rods had been sewn into them. By the following morning, they would revive a little, feeling more flexible, most of the visceral sensation having dissipated.

As throughout chemotherapy, I continued with twice-weekly sessions of acupuncture. Niccala had worked on my legs to bring some energy back to them as she had done when I was undergoing chemo, but this time her initial treatments were not working; then she got it right – not with needles but with lots of moxa. My legs were far from normality, but they revived sufficiently for me to be confident that I would still be able to walk at the end of radiotherapy. In particular, Niccala had dispelled the physical sensation of 'dread' from my traumatized muscles, enabling me to make the few steps each day absolutely necessary to a sense of relative independence.

Prostrate prostate and the battle of the bladder

But the radiation was affecting more than just my legs; my prostate gland was under daily onslaught so that passing and holding water were increasingly toilsome.

One day, my treatment was significantly delayed as Venus was on holiday and Mars had a hiccup. Like several others, I had already drunk the required amount of water and my bladder was expanding at a worrying rate. A growing queue of men sat tight, some with their legs perhaps uncharacteristically crossed, maybe wondering why the current patient was taking so long.

But it was not just men who had to hold their water; women receiving radiotherapy to the pelvis also underwent a similar preparation.

'You're a bit overfull', one of my radiographers informed me, with typical English understatement, when my turn eventually came. 'Could you pass some water without letting it *all* go?'

'I doubt it… Is it too full for treatment?'

'Only if you can't hang on to it.'

'Then let's do it.' They quickly positioned me then left. Immediately, I regretted my decision. I had just wanted to get the treatment over quickly, but I was struggling to hold on, worried that my bladder might suddenly expel its contents without my consent.

(What *are* they up to in there?) They seemed to be taking an age to make their final adjustments.

'Sorry, mate. We've had enough of this', my bladder complained. 'Me and the muscles are constantly being abused and overworked… We're going on strike.'

'No, no; please don't. Honestly, I won't drink another drop today!'

'Should've thought about that before, guv.'

A sudden, slight movement of the table. (Hope at last.)

'But it's only a matter of seconds, now…'

'No use, mate, we're running out of power.'

Yet more delay. (For heaven's sake, come on!)

'No use calling out to that lot; they can't hear yer.'

A sudden thud.

'It's about to start!'

'Oh yeah? …We're about to stop.'

'No, no! Not now! The beam will hit my intestine if you quit now.'

'Not our problem, mate. Demarcation.'

'What?!'

'Not our job pushing your inflated, fat-cat intestine out of the way.'

The long awaited and overdue buzz commenced as merciful Mercury spun into orbit.

'Okay lads… LET GO!'

'Christ!'

*

The radiographers got me off the table quickly when they came back. 'You can pass water here, if you like', one of them said a little apologetically, handing me a disposable urinal.

'No. Just let me get to the loo fast.' As quickly as my quaking legs could carry me, miraculously replenished with fresh energy, gown swinging open at the back Cyril-style, I darted into the Ladies opposite where I experienced the bliss of release.

'That was a close call', I commented to Sangita, after changing out of my gown. 'Don't know how I managed to hang on.'

'Yes, it's a problem as the treatment progresses… I sometimes think we ask too much of patients.' Hmm… 'But you'll get through it', she said smiling encouragingly.

Once, previously, as she had been about to usher me into the changing room, she had exclaimed, 'Whoops! Someone's had an accident... Would you be okay changing in the treatment room?'

'Sure.'

Now I could better understand the significance of the occasional damp patch on the changing-room chair... And Cyril's merry dance. I had not yet had a spill, but at times it had been very close. And it's not just water. When the nearest toilet is occupied and the enema insists on further, immediate evacuation, what is a man to do? Spin his wheels with Herculean strength to the next, even if it's the Ladies.

6

Susie and the Skunk

I had intended to visit Jayamitra, who was dying at St Joseph's Hospice in East London, stricken by the same disease that was afflicting me, but my legs were so weak it would have cost a huge effort to get there. He died before they had regained their strength.

Unfortunately for him, like many men, he had not been diagnosed until well after his cancer had metastasized. So far, I had been lucky; though at a relatively advanced stage, mine was still potentially curable at the time of diagnosis. But it had probably been a close call.

'What's going on with you guys?' an old friend had asked, referring to the number of Order members recently diagnosed with prostate cancer. 'I've had my PSA levels tested every year since I was fifty.'

But, you see, 'Most men die *with* prostate cancer, not *of* it' is the common refrain, which is meant to reassure and was voiced to me even by a GP. Doubtless it is true, but it can trivialize a serious disease, perhaps obscuring the fact that prostate cancer now kills more men than breast cancer kills women.

It would never have occurred to me to have requested an annual PSA test from my GP. Had I done so, as some of my friends had, I might have spared myself and my friends a lot of inconvenience. I might not now be facing the threat to my life that confronts me daily, and I would have saved the NHS a huge amount of money. Let my fate be a warning to any man reading this.

Having pursued a healthy lifestyle and having enjoyed robust health all my life, perhaps unconsciously I had considered myself immune to any form of cancer. Moreover, I had believed that there had been no family history. Then, five years before my diagnosis, I learned that my paternal grandmother had succumbed to breast cancer, not to diabetes as I had previously understood.

More recently I learned that a link has been established between breast and prostate cancer. So that any man who has a close female relative who developed breast cancer might be more susceptible to prostate cancer. (I believe that this also works in reverse.)

But, whatever the cause, it did not change the reality I had been made to face as, once more, I lay on Mercury's altar, offering up my cancer cells to his devouring beam.

More water wars

Even before I had finally made it into the treatment room, I knew there would be further delay.

'Craig gone for the bladder scanner?'

'Yeah', Sangita replied. Why had I bothered to ask? I had seen that wretched, wayward planet-hopper heading for Saturn just a few minutes earlier. It's never there when a bladder is getting inflated ideas of its own importance.

The department had two scanners, but one had been unserviceable ever since I began my treatment, leaving the other to be shared by the entire solar system. Often, I had lain on the table straining my ears for the slightest hint of rattling wheels, heralding its approach from some remote celestial body. Frequently I had been beguiled by phantom sounds of that longed-for clattering along the corridor that promised imminent relief, only to be disappointed, duped again by an auditory hallucination conjured by my wishful imagination.

'Are you sure you don't want to empty?' Sangita asked, with a hint of anxiety when Craig read the scan reading. Of course! But not until after the treatment.

'Let's go. Just be quick.' They promised – and they were. They raced through the usual protocol asking me for my address and date of birth before double-checking my dosage.

'Two loops at 1.2 volts', Craig said. Sangita confirmed. He had spoken softly as always, as if I was not supposed to hear, but, living with a medical engineer, I now knew that that meant *megavolts*. Jeepers! First they poison you with chemo, then they fry you. Not that the megavolts actually hit you, but it takes that much power to generate the radiation that does.

'Here… in case you need it.' A seemingly disembodied hand appeared and a soft grey object was thrust onto my chest by Sangita. I clutched it with both hands, which had been clasped together high on my chest, corpse-style – as if interred within some sepulchral chamber – well out of the way of the beam's path. I laughed when I recognized the urinal.

'Thanks… but I won't.'

Then the bleeping warned of the closing door as I heard the scurry of her retreating steps overlaid by her familiar, brief valediction, 'Nice and still… Here we go!' And the wall of lead closed on me, sealing me within, like the boulder in front of Christ's tomb, alone once more at the heart of Mercury's orbit, bracing myself for the latest battle with that bloated water bag. All the whingeing and whining going on in my nether regions was so unfair. It really was not my fault that it was all but brimming. Mercury had been uncooperative so that again things were running late, and my bladder was more than thirty minutes fuller than it should have been.

'Thank you for being so patient', Craig said, somewhat guiltily, as soon as they returned.

'Oh, it's not your fault', I insisted, removing the tissue they had placed as usual (in the absence of fig leaves readily at hand) to cover my exposed genitals. 'Here – you can keep it', I said to Sangita, after hitching up my boxer shorts, as I returned the urinal to her. 'Forgive me, but I'm heading straight for the Ladies.'

'Please feel free!' she responded, smiling encouragingly. It was reassuring to have official sanction. Drat! It was engaged; fortunately, the Gents was not. As nonchalantly as I could, I sauntered along, desperate to keep face, holding the back of my gown closed as I headed for my distant destination, close to Mars.

What Sangita nicked

The following morning, I had a bit less in my bladder – not that it refrained from its inveterate grumbling.

As I returned to change out of my gown in one of the two cubicles, the door of the other was wide open. A man, probably in his forties, was sitting there gowned and highly agitated. He could keep neither his arms nor his feet still, the latter tap-dancing the floor. I smiled encouragement into his anxious eyes, but he didn't seem to register my presence. He was obviously uncomfortably full.

'You can come through now', I heard the familiar voice of Sangita call out to him, as I closed the cubicle door behind me, mercifully glad that I had only nine more dates with Mercury. Many times had I waited with anticipation for the sound of Sangita's voice uttering those same words to usher me in.

A few days later, as I was about to lie down ready for the beam, I noticed a swish bladder scanner nearby. 'You've got a new one!'

'Yeah', Sangita replied.

'So now you have two working machines again.'

'No… We nicked this one from the CT unit. It'll have to go back.'

'Oh… pity.' I pondered a moment before putting a question that had troubled me for a while. 'Has anyone ever passed water during treatment?'

'It happens – more often than you might think', Rick responded.

'Not that I'm about to, by the way!' I said, reassuring myself as much as him, as he scanned my bladder.

'Well, if you're able to hold less and less, start doing the pelvic-floor exercises again', he advised.

'Oh, I never did them; I could hold 700 mils before starting all this.'

'Really… You're a bit over', he said checking the reading. 'If you can hold this much at this stage, you'll be fine.' Good – but it was costing more and more effort, especially at night. If I woke up with what felt like a full bladder, passing water was strenuous and could take several minutes. It was as if my muscles were still asleep; some were waking up rather grumpily, convulsing as if I was about to vomit.

Dependent

Several people who had undergone both chemo and radiotherapy had told me that the latter was much easier. I could understand that, but, in some respects, I had found it much more difficult. The fatigue in my legs had never been so severe under chemo and my strength had always recovered significantly as each cycle wore on. But with radiotherapy there was little respite. During the final weeks of my treatment, I had a three-day break due to a bank holiday, and by the end I felt the energy returning, which was heartening.

'You'll be surprised how quickly it will return when you've finished', Rick had assured me when I mentioned it to him.

In the meantime, however, I had become markedly dependent on others, and was wheelchair-bound if not housebound. Getting up the two flights of stairs to my room from the front door had become increasingly taxing, and occasionally I needed to be virtually carried up as I had strained the muscles on my upper arms. Pushing myself upstairs with my arms several times a day, together with spinning my wheels over-enthusiastically, had taken its toll.

'Have you used a wheelchair before?' one of the radiotherapy receptionists had asked me.

'No.'

'But you seem remarkably adept.' Perhaps I had been, but now I could barely propel myself forward!

*

At least I had sufficient energy to get downstairs to the LBC, though not as frequently as I would have liked. On one occasion, during this period, I spoke about Amoghasiddhi, an archetypal Buddha figure who had always had great personal appeal because of his association with the virtue of fearlessness. Unfortunately, I had been feeling particularly fatigued. Perhaps I should have found a stand-in, but I was inspired by the unobstructed success associated with his name and, as ever, I had been reluctant to throw away the opportunity.

Susie and me

Sometimes I had wondered about Susie and what might have passed through *her* mind, her memory haunting the recesses of mine. At the very beginning, the same parasite had been my agent and hers. I had worked with her at the Octagon Theatre in Bolton long before she received her BAFTA and Tony Award nominations. I had lost track of her when I stopped working as an actor, but I heard of her occasionally from mutual friends.

She had worked to the last, seemingly denying it – though all her friends knew – and she refused to talk about it or acknowledge it, they said. She was only thirty-four, same age as me – then. I was saddened when I heard – and shocked. Albert Finney had hosted her memorial programme at the National Theatre. She was the first person I knew who had died of cancer.

I would never deny my cancer, either to myself or to others – even if that is what *she* did – although I find it difficult to believe that she would have denied it to herself, and I could understand if she had refused to talk about it with others, perhaps defiantly so. I had known from the outset that my cancer could kill me, as it still could, but I did not care to dwell on the details and only spoke about them reluctantly.

And yet, did that not convict me of a subtler form of the same crime? Had not her memory returned to accuse me? So often I was unwilling to get too close to the edge, not wanting to look into the abyss, even though when I had done so it had vitalized me, focusing my mind on the deeper issues I had wanted to confront. Occasionally I had been dragged there by circumstance – a chance comment, the glance of fear or repulsion in someone's eyes – and was forced to stand and look down once more.

Initially, I had just wanted to get through the treatment then deal with the outcome when it was over – so I had convinced myself. But that was merely a rationalization of the reluctance I was unwilling to acknowledge, an avoidance tactic to prevent me from uncovering what lay beneath the resistance. But there comes a time…

Prognosis

My treatment was virtually over. It was my final visit to Mercury, but first I had to see my consultant. 'I'm sorry to have kept you waiting so long', she said. 'I had wanted to call you in earlier, but I was hijacked by another patient.'

I wheeled myself into the consulting room. 'I'm a bit concerned to see you in that wheelchair', she said; her words were heartfelt, not merely dutiful. We had developed a good rapport, and I had come to like and appreciate her.

'Oh, I can walk', I assured her, 'but not very far'. She then introduced me to her latest registrar and I wondered: are there any male prostate-cancer specialists? I have yet to meet one. I must ask her next time.

After a few pleasantries, we then got down to serious matters. 'There's a fifty per cent chance that the cancer will recur', she began. 'You see, once it gets into the lymphatic system, it is very difficult to cure', she continued, looking me straight in the eye as I returned her gaze. 'We'll monitor you every six months', she said, handing me a slip for my next blood test, six weeks hence, before our next consultation.

My blessed lymph nodes! I had always known that they were the most dangerous factor in my diagnosis: 'T3b N1 M0 Gleason 4+5=9'. 'N1' referred to the lymph nodes; 'M0' indicated that the cancer had not travelled beyond the pelvis, meaning that it was still curable. N1 was my potential assassin; M0 had been my saviour, up until now. This was only just the right side of terminal illness; had M0 been M1, I would now be heading rapidly towards the bardo of death, driven hard by my 4+5 tumour – speeding, in fact, like a car hurtling recklessly along a motorway well beyond the speed limit, indifferent to whatever was caught in its way, bent on self-destruction.

How unpredictable is life! Several years ago, Bhante had been listening to the radio, as he often did. During one programme, he had heard it claimed that one in four of my generation could expect to live to be a hundred. He later grinned, wagging his finger at me; 'And you will be one of them', he said firmly, as if he had no doubt. The thought horrified me, having witnessed the reality of old age, but the chances of that happening now must be slim, whatever they may have been in the past. If I survive this disease, I will consider myself to have been truly blessed.

'I'd like you to help me make a financial decision', I said to the consultant. 'By having deferred my state pension, I have two options – I can accept either a rise or a lump sum, but to take the increase only makes sense if I have a good chance of living another seven years.' She looked at me seriously. 'If I'm likely to be dead in three years' time, I would opt for the lump sum… You can work out the question.'

'You mean, if I was to place a bet, which would I choose?'

'Yes.'

'I'd put my money on the first; I think you have a *very* good chance of living another seven years', she said, smiling.

She then arranged a DEXA scan for me, as I had now been on leuprorelin for almost nine months. As my mother had had osteoporosis, it was possible that this treatment would reduce my bone density, in which case I would need to take a calcium supplement. I was already benefiting from hot flushes, courtesy of my twelve-weekly injections, but, thankfully, the man boobs had not manifested. I am still able to hold my head high at the swimming pool.

Farewell

It was late afternoon by the time I headed for Mercury. 'I've got something for you', said Rick.

'And I have something for you, too', I replied; 'I'll give it to you when I come through.' He handed me a flier for a session on 'health and well-being for men with prostate cancer, post treatment'. 'Thanks, but I don't think I'll come.' After changing into a gown, I passed once more beyond that impenetrable barrier that would soon close on me for the last time.

'Here', I said, handing over my gift together with a card and a flier, 'this is for all of you.' He smiled warmly, then set me up for my final treatment. There was just enough water in my bladder to start straight away; soon afterwards, Mercury orbited me and I was done.

Another dry run – not that I had ever seriously thought I might leak – despite having undergone thirty-nine sessions. I had only met one other patient prescribed that many; everyone else had been scheduled for twenty-nine, or much less. Even ambulance drivers were astonished that I had so many appointments.

When I came out of the cubicle, having changed out of the gown, Rick was waiting for me extending his hand, obviously wanting more than just to shake mine; but we were men and I was almost old enough to be his grandfather. Although we bungled it, there could be no mistaking the mutual warmth as we wished each other well.

'Thanks for this', he said, still grasping the flier advertising the LBC open day I had given him. He seemed interested and knew that I would probably be present the following Sunday, even though I would not be teaching.

I was sad to say goodbye; I had liked him from the start, when he had spoken at the introductory radiotherapy seminar, and we had often had brief chats since – as I had also with Yasmin. I was sorry not to be able to say a few parting words both to her and to Sangita – who had been with me for almost every treatment.

*

Although I was glad to have both chemotherapy and radiotherapy behind me, as I left Mercury I felt a sudden, brief surge of insecurity and immediately understood why. While undergoing these radical treatments, there is a sense that the cancer is under control – that for the time being you are unlikely to deteriorate – and you are in regular contact with people who are looking after you; then the treatment is suddenly over. Having been seduced into a false sense of security, you are now forced to remember that you are on your own – as you always have been.

> *Oh build your ship of death, oh build it!*
> *for you will need it.*
> *For the voyage of oblivion awaits you.*[6]

I had acted long ago on Lawrence's exhortation, but had kept to harbour. Even so, in the moment, I felt I had launched into stormy seas, a solitary sailor in a small boat, seeking the deep calm beyond.

Nutters

I had the car to myself as I was driven back from the hospital by the African driver. The radio was on, as usual, and there was the hourly pause in the music for the latest news. I was barely conscious of the disembodied, deadpan voice seemingly recounting the same old stories, until I heard, with a mixture of amusement and horrified dismay, that 'The Poundland chain announced today that it is withdrawing one of its products, out of concerns that it may be offensive to people with mental-health issues. As from today, packets of chocolate-coated peanuts, marketed as "Nutters", will be removed from shelves…'

The driver doubled up in a fit of uncontrollable laughter. Fortunately, we were stationary, locked in a traffic jam. When he had recovered, I grinned at him. 'I'm glad you find that funny', I said.

He shook his head. 'Man… Oh man!' he exclaimed; he continued to chuckle, while I inwardly asked myself, 'Who are the *real* nutters?'

Recur?

It was a black card, on which the letters had been printed in large blue type: *'Urgent'*. Beneath, in smaller white characters, it said, *'I have a medical condition that means I need to use a toilet quickly. Please can you help?'* I had never used it and could not imagine I ever would, but it had been inside my wallet ever since it had been given to me at the radiotherapy seminar. 'Just go into any pub, show it to them, and they'll let you use the toilet', Rick had said. Apparently, local-government authorities were paying the celebrated alehouses of England for this service – it is cheaper than funding public toilets.

I had never taken note of the words on the reverse side of the card, but I did now: *'Speak to our Specialist Nurses'*, it urged and so, since a question had surfaced since my consultation the previous day, I called the Prostate Cancer UK helpline. What was the significance of the word 'recur'?

'It could recur within five years locally or remotely', the nurse said, confirming what I had suspected. 'Remotely' would mean secondary tumours and terminal illness. Then *she* had questions for *me*, which I was happy to answer. I told her about my treatment, since she asked.

'Then you're lucky', she said. 'You're one of the first to receive this sequence. Although it is early days, studies suggest that this may significantly reduce the likelihood of recurrence. If it does recur, there's always docetaxel', she continued, as if that might reassure me. 'You're a responder; not everybody is.' Good – but I doubted that I would be willing to endure a second round of chemo, should the worst happen.

After further questions, we discussed the fatigue in my legs. She was not surprised; she had encountered it several times before.

'Because the cancer got into your lymphatic system, that will have been heavily targeted by your treatment. That's why they gave you thirty-nine sessions of teletherapy. The lymph glands release fluid to your muscles, which helps you to walk, but yours have been pounded very hard to get rid of the cancer. Don't expect the energy to come back quickly. It could take quite a while.'

A funeral

Later that day I went to Jayamitra's funeral. I had thought twice about attending, as my legs were feeling particularly weak, and had decided not to go. But how could I not? He was my Dharma brother.

He had always seemed to have held me in good regard, occasionally sending me cards of appreciation, from which it was evident that he felt an affinity with me. We had also lived together for a few months fourteen years previously and, poignantly, we had met twice at the hospital where we had both been treated for a common disease to which he had succumbed at last.

Seeing his body in the LBC shrine room was a strong reminder of the perilous situation I was in. Messengers of death seemed to be approaching me from several directions at once and, though I did not yet know it, another was fast approaching.

The old skunk

It was still only twenty-four hours since I had talked with my consultant, but so intense had been the interval between our consultation and the end of the funeral that time seemed to have been suspended. Yet I had had precious few moments to reflect. All my mental energy had been engaged by the tumult that had erupted in my mind as I was cast into the confusion of riotous, conflicting mental states. And still no respite seemed in sight.

The turbulence I was experiencing was reminiscent of a two-month period during the early part of a nine-month solitary retreat four years previously, but, on that occasion, of course, there had been nobody to whom I could talk to help me clarify what was happening. I had been thrown hard against my inner resources, even to the point of feeling that I was in danger of losing my mind. I had had to fight extremely hard to come out on top.

This was the key experience that had enabled me, right from the start, to deal positively with cancer. It had been the rehearsal before the real show. On that earlier occasion, I had been dealing with phantoms, but the spectre haunting me now had more substance and I knew that I must take a step further.

Trying to understand what I was actually feeling had become a conundrum – it seemed so complex. I needed to objectify the turmoil that this succession of events had precipitated. Fortunately, at its height, I had the perfect opportunity, just a few hours after the funeral. It was 'community night' – the one time each week when, after the usual shared meal and household chores, the men I live with and I spend the remainder of the evening together.

They listened patiently and sympathetically as I recounted the ferment that was stirring within, and when I had finished they all seemed at a loss for words – not that I expected any – but they had done what was required; their willingness to listen had helped me to perceive the more obscure currents within my mind, highlighting the individual conflicts pummelling its equilibrium.

What *was* I feeling? It was still hard to tell, but something had loosened. The previous night, all I had felt was a tight knot in my abdomen. Fear seemed the obvious culprit. I knew that fear was a protective mask worn by self-clinging – a facade to keep threats at bay. I had seen it before. 'Stand back!' it seemed to say, 'you are entering dangerous territory.' But it was a face, with no living feature, attached above a scarecrow's fluttering rags, hiding a powerful force I had, perhaps, once glimpsed, but that dared not be seen by human eye. How easy it was to be taken in by its masquerade then rapidly retreat, like a rabbit startled by a rustle in the grass, diving deep into the darkness of its warren, terror-stricken.

No; it was not fear – at least not predominantly, if at all. It was something closer to the surface. Shock, perhaps? No, something else. I knew the sensation. It was painfully familiar, then slowly it revealed itself. Companion to Despair, I finally recognized the stench of that old skunk, Loss. It seemed absurd; I had lost nothing, but here it was, fouling my mind, dogging me like a professional mourner at a funeral. 'Thank you for coming… Now you may leave.'

And yet… I had a sense that my life was over – not that I was about to die, but that I was leaving my old life behind for good. Whatever might await me in the future was seemingly more unpredictable than ever – a sensation I felt all the more acutely when I heard that the cancer of an old friend, who had had the same diagnosis as me, had just recurred.

Perhaps, perhaps…

I had been in danger of losing perspective by reacting against uncertainty. But cancer *is* uncertainty; samsara is uncertainty. Why do I find it so difficult to welcome it? Does it not lead to unexpected adventure, to the new experience that revitalizes me? Is it not ultimately my friend?

How contrary I am! I did not want reassurance, yet I had sought it. I did not wish for hope, yet I had pursued it. In the circumstances, I had not yet sufficiently seen the vanity of either, though I knew they were both empty and that neither could deliver anything other than a hardening of the deeply engrained habit I sought to break down. At such moments, I would invoke the spirit of Vajrapani to stiffen my resolve. One impulse had been pitched hard against another. I had tried to resist the forces that led to comfort and to endure the discomfort of their absence. Hence this impasse, this terrible, tightening knot in my belly, which at last was unravelling to leave me in peace.

I was content. And so I should be – my hair was growing. 'It suits you. You should keep it like that', they kept saying. 'You're looking really well' was the other refrain, nearly always accompanied with such big smiles. I had looked yellow; I had looked grey, they had said; but not any more.

And don't believe everything they tell you about these treatments. I had solemnly signed my consent in the presence of a beautiful young woman. Before she had permitted me to do so, she had warned that radiotherapy would make me impotent – not that it might, but that it *would*. I was rather pleased about that. Unfortunately, it failed. My erectile function has survived the severest nuking medical practice permits, albeit with less power than I had been accustomed to. And I now have another reason, should I have needed one, not to invest in a vacuum pump.

I may yet live to be a hundred. If there is a fifty per cent chance of my cancer recurring, there must surely be an equal possibility it will not. At the very least, I have been given a stay of execution, so far as cancer is concerned – perhaps even a new lease of life. Hmm... perhaps.

The greatest blessing

But something new had emerged. When I had been diagnosed with hypertension on my sixty-seventh birthday I was shocked. This sort of thing did not, *should not*, happen to me, but it had. It was the first time that I had had to face a serious health issue. Then I saw that old skunk, tail up, head turned, taking aim, mischief in its eye, about to squirt. Vainly I ran for cover, then I mourned.

I had something substantial to offer others, I believed. I had been blessed when young by a spiritual friend of great depth and substance. It had taken decades for his blessing to mature, but, if my health failed, its potential benefit to others would be lost.

Eighteen months later, I knew I had a serious cancer; eleven months more and the treatment was over. It was then that I felt most keenly and urgently not so much that I wanted to live (though, of course, I do) but that I had a duty to live as long as I could – even to a hundred years, or more (perish the thought). I must preserve and cherish the blessing I have received and pass it on to others. I have little else to live for, but that is quite something.

A young man recently came to see me. We had talked several months previously in a chance encounter in Victoria Park one beautiful spring day, while I was still in the midst of chemo. He had heard me speak about my experience of cancer at the LBC, and he had his own tragic tale to tell.

Now it was autumn, and he told me that I had become an important figure in his life because of my 'mature' attitude in the face of cancer and death. He had never encountered that before, he said, though he had sought it. For him, I had become an exemplar. May I not fail him – or anybody else. May I truly become a beacon for others.

7

Living Paradoxes

'Are you bored?' he asked. I was sitting quietly reflecting after breakfast, and was startled by the question.

'Why should I be bored?'

'Well, you know, all this time you've not been able to do very much.' True, but I was never bored. I cannot remember the last time I was significantly bored. Yes, sometimes I had been bored with a film I was watching or with a particular conversation, but generally bored? No. I don't get bored. Chemotherapy, for example, is far from boring; it's exciting – unpleasant, I grant you, sometimes wearing, but never boring. Although I had wearied of it a little towards the end – I confess – I had cast off my weariness quickly.

I would wish them on no one, but the treatments I had received had opened up new experience to me in many ways, thereby enriching my life.

Most unforeseen, perhaps, was a much deeper appreciation of Beethoven's late string quartets. Often, while undergoing chemo, I had very little energy for anything, and I lay for hours listening to music. I was living a paradox, simultaneously experiencing the travails of an ailing body, like a swan grounded by a broken wing, while yet being uplifted by the most sublime music, a vulture riding a thermal to the heavens and beyond.

I listened to the quartets countless times, their strains seeping into me, penetrating further and further. Perhaps not so surprising: they were Beethoven's swansong. There seems to be a profound poignancy suffusing the slower movements, especially his 'Song of thanksgiving to the Divinity' (on recovery from serious illness). Did I feel a spiritual kinship with the genius of the music, a solidarity with its source?

Recurrence

A few weeks after my final radiotherapy session, I had to return to see my dermatologist for a routine check. The carcinoma that had been removed in India had recurred a year later and had required further treatment.

'It looks beautiful to me', the dermatologist said, referring to the long, smooth surgical scar on my arm, now no longer blemished by cancer cells. At last it had gone.

'Hospitals seem to be becoming my home from home', I said.

'Well that's not good, is it?'

I shook my head. 'Could I be discharged, please?'

She agreed. 'If anything recurs, let your GP know and we'll see you within two weeks.'

The NHS can be truly wonderful.

Lymphatic reaction

Excessive optimism frequently leads me into trouble. Ten days after being utterly dependent on a wheelchair, I sent it packing. And that was just three days after being stranded a few hundred metres from the LBC without the energy to walk back. Muditasri had had to return for my wheelchair. Even so, I was already back in the pool training, as I had enough energy to walk there and back.

'It got into my lymphatic system', I was explaining to a fellow swimmer, and could proceed no further as his reaction was instantaneous.

'Oh, I know what *that* means!' he said with an involuntary shudder, triggering a shiver in my mind, his eyes shrinking back with fear. The power of words is truly extraordinary. By now I was impervious to such reactions and the echoes they sound within my mind. He had asked how I was, and I had told him. I had been urging him, ever since I had been diagnosed, to get a PSA test, as he was clearly at risk: his father had metastatic prostate cancer.

'You don't want to end up like me', I said firmly, smiling encouragement. That finally seemed to galvanize him.

'Well, maybe I will.' Later he thanked me for nagging him. His GP arranged an early hospital appointment after they got the results.

I don't know why I had pressed him about this. In a sense it was none of my business; I barely knew him other than as a friendly presence in the changing room, yet I felt urged to do it. I had not suggested to anyone else that they get tested. However, it transpired that he too had a stage 3b tumour. Whenever we bump into each other now he is always pleased to see me, evidently very grateful. Perhaps, had it not been for me, his diagnosis would have come too late for his life to be spared.

It's always raining...

And of course, I was back on my bike. I should have read the signs. I was getting cocky. One day I cycled seven miles; the following day I swam 900 metres; on the third day I did the same, swimming harder – and walked over 10,000 steps, according to my fitness tracker. On the fourth day, when I got out of bed I could hardly stand.

That was problematic. I had to get a train late that afternoon to Manchester to participate in the stone-setting ceremony for Dayanatha's late father, and I was determined to go. I was touched to have been asked to attend, and pleased to have this opportunity to strengthen our growing friendship.

I travelled to Euston station by the Underground, helped by Prajnamanas. The following day, Sunday, was cold, windy, and wet – Manchester! But that was not why it was tough. Although everyone else was standing in the packed chapel at the cemetery, I sat at one side throughout the service as standing taxes me even more than walking.

When the rabbi had finished, Dayanatha spoke movingly about his father; afterwards, I stood with Prajnamanas by the door, leaning against the wall to take some of the weight off my feet, holding a box with stones for people to take and put on top of the gravestone. Amused to think it *très cardinalesque*, I had chosen a scarlet kippa, but it sat precariously on my head and I was now anxious lest it might take flight with the gusting wind. I did not remove it, as I was uncertain of the protocol and did not wish to risk offence.

'Thank you so much for coming', Dayanatha's elderly grandmother said to me as she came out, 'it means so much to him.' Her words were echoed by his mother. Their warmth took the chill out of the wind and I was glad that I had come, despite having to stand for the ceremony at the graveside on tremulous limbs, and despite my frantic attempts to secure my flighty kippa.

The following day, I had an acupuncture appointment. 'I think I might have overdone it a bit', I confessed as I shambled through the door. Niccala laughed, then later admonished me. I must conserve my energy at least until the new year, she insisted.

I had never seriously considered that I would need to convalesce. I am not used to being ill and, because the cancer itself had caused me no pain, it was difficult to believe that my body was diseased. I did not disbelieve that I had a tumour, but I had never seen or felt it. I had taken my diagnosis on trust, and had therefore consented to treatment. Experientially, however, I was recovering from the therapies, not cancer, and it was difficult for me to grasp that *that* warranted convalescence. But, at last, I understood… I think.

*

The enervation, however, was not just physical. With the onset of chemo, I had stopped meditating because the mental fatigue was so extreme. I had hoped to pick up my daily practice when chemo was over, but my lethargy continued throughout radiotherapy, albeit less severely. For seven months I had not meditated, and yet my emotional positivity had sustained itself throughout and at times my mental acuity was as sharp as ever. This would have been impossible without forty-five years of continuous Dharma practice (including daily meditation) behind me, but, even so, I did not wish to become complacent and was eager to re-establish my routine. In the weeks following my treatment I gradually succeeded.

Remission

Six weeks had passed since I had finished radiotherapy, and I had returned to the hospital for yet another encounter with a phlebotomist.

Two days later came my final consultation. Thereafter I would only return for six-monthly reviews preceded by a blood test.

'How are you?' my consultant asked.

'*I'm* always very well', I replied, 'it's this wretched body that's the problem.' Indeed; still, I really ought to resist this stale joke, which I have used far too often... but it is so tempting; it usually provokes a chuckle – as it did on this occasion. 'I really need a new one', I continued. 'Not that

I intend to do anything about that, by the way', I hastily added.

'I'm relieved to see you out of that wheelchair', she said, trying to get serious. 'I was very worried about that. Had you turned up in one this time I would have had to give you something that would have made you *really* sick.'

'You've already done that', I quipped.

No more nonsense – to business.

'Your blood results were excellent. Your PSA is down to 0.003. That's an extremely good result at this stage', she said with typical enthusiasm when communicating something positive. A quick mental calculation: it had been roughly 15,000 times more than that when I began.

'Is that the hormone therapy?'

'No. Radiotherapy. The last time we tested it, it was 1.42 when you were still on chemo. It was 43 before you started treatment.'

'According to my GP it was 46', I insisted (wrongly, I discovered later), not wanting to be cheated by one iota of the seriousness of my diagnosis – there's status in this. Another quick calculation: 1.42 is approximately 473 times more than my current level – a further huge shift. 'So if I'm asked, for legal purposes, "Do you have cancer?", what is the most truthful answer?'

'For insurance, "Yes".'

'What's my actual status?'

'You're in remission.'

'What does that mean?'

'There's no evidence of cancer present anywhere in your body at the moment.'

*

So I was given a reprieve until my first review, six months later. I must live my life in biannual cycles, never forgetting those last three words – *at the moment* – mindful that I may be living merely on borrowed time, and that the cancer might already have returned even when her words were spoken. It can recur very quickly.

My life remained on the line, as it had been for a year since I was first diagnosed, yet I forget so quickly and easily, like a man on death row who cannot believe his executioner will ever call.

'Don't you ever wake up scared in the middle of the night?' one of my friends had asked. Never. The thought of cancer does not disturb my dreams any more than my waking life. It used to scare me *before* afflicting me; now that it threatens my life, it no longer does. How perverse. It's simply the reality I face. I'm no more or less conscious of it than I am of the sun when it shines. It is only at relatively rare moments, usually in conversation, that I'm conscious of cancer – and then only fleetingly, mostly free from disquiet. Then begins the struggle to overcome my wilful ignorance, to seize the moment of awareness, daring to stand on the edge and look down, perhaps to soar above the abyss.

Possibly I lack imagination – how could I *not* be afraid of it? I cannot answer my own question. Probably I should be shot through with shivers of fear – it's a terrible, painful disease – but I am not. What I fear most is dying with a mind deadened by morphine, with its concomitant confusion. I am determined to greet the Grim Reaper with a bright mind, and will take any steps necessary to ensure that I do.

*

'Are there any other lingering side effects from the radio-therapy?' my consultant continued. I could think of none, other than the fatigue, having forgotten, in the moment, my chronically dry left eye. But what about my bones?

'There's a slight thinning; you don't have osteoporosis but osteopenia, which can lead to it. It's too early for leuprorelin to have caused that.' She prescribed calcium and vitamin D. 'You may be able to come off the hormone therapy after two years instead of three.' These were soothing words to one whose manly breast was under threat. 'I'll let you know when we have the results of the latest studies.' May the gods preserve my chest – a perfect plateau blighted by neither hill nor dale.

'I still have neuropathy in my hands and feet.'

'That may take between eighteen months and two years to clear. Chemo destroys the nerve endings; they take a while to grow back.' She paused before continuing. 'You may not see me the next time you come', she explained. 'The nurses may be taking over the reviews of patients in remission – a change I'm trying to resist, but I may not be able to do so much longer.'

'Well, I hope I *do* see you', I said with feeling, saddened by her disclosure. 'I'm grateful for everything you've done for me.' When you have a good rapport with a doctor, you want that relationship to continue. Though we had had our differences over acupuncture, it had been evident from our first meeting that she took a genuine interest in her patients – certainly, she did so with me. I had felt immediately at ease with her bright, lively personality, and had always found her warm, sympathetic, good-humoured – and candid when necessary.

Suddenly I was conscious that I had no gift for her. I had wanted to give her something at the end of radiotherapy – but what? The chocolates I had given to my radiographers and the receptionists would be hopelessly inadequate given how indebted I felt.

How do you adequately thank someone who may have saved your life? In context, that may sound overblown. Had she not simply done her job, for which she is well paid? Perhaps. But there is a human dimension that can easily be overlooked and undervalued. We had a positive and effective relationship characterized by the trust that should arise naturally between doctors and patients, but which often does not. I imagine that mental attitudes on both sides of the clinical divide might have a bearing on the outcome of treatment.

Even if this thing finally kills me – even were it to do so relatively quickly – I'm sure that I shall continue to feel greatly indebted to her, grateful at least for the stay of execution she has given me from the ravages of cancer, grateful for prolonging my much-valued opportunity to give of my experience to those who esteem it. However, it is vital not just to *feel* gratitude, but to *express* it. Whatever stirrings of positive emotion one feels should be encouraged and acted on, as this strengthens it and weakens its negative counterpart. I knew from experience that this attitude had helped me displace my bad habits with good. But, perhaps more significantly, countless times I had seen the positive effects on others of voicing a few words of appreciation.

On the present occasion, I felt I had been fortunate, but I did not know how to express my upsurge of gratitude appropriately – until fortune intervened.

Sir Antony

Antony Gormley came to the LBC to be interviewed by Maitreyabandhu as part of his *Poetry East* programme. As usual, it was a wonderful evening. Who else other than Maitreyabandhu could have pulled it off? I sat next to his fellow poet and poetry mentor, Mimi Khalvati. 'I don't know how he does it', she said. 'His preparation is so thorough. There's nothing else like this on the literary scene. What he does is unique.'

Antony Gormley is a sculptor, of course, not a poet, and he's almost a Buddhist. Afterwards he signed books, including the Phaidon book on his work. 'Could you dedicate this to "Angela"?' I asked. He readily agreed.

During the interview, he had spoken very warmly about the north-east of England – its culture, landscape, and people – even mentioning my home town.

'By the way, I was born in Middlesbrough just after the war', I said, after he had signed the book. His face lit up. 'My father was a fitter in the shipyards.'

I might have been an old and cherished friend, given the warmth with which he put his arm around me. (What a shameless fraud I am, given my ambivalence to my birthplace.) He was evidently about to launch eagerly into some discourse about the north-east, which, sadly, I had to check, as there was a long queue of people behind me awaiting his signature. Nonetheless, I now had the perfect gift.

Two days later, I left the book at the hospital with a card and a letter of appreciation. Both the book and my words were warmly received.

*

Now that I was evidently looking well, several people told me how dreadful I had looked, especially towards the end of my treatment. One of my friends had even thought that I was not going to survive it, though others seemed to think I was much worse than I ever felt – a dead man walking, as one had put it to me.

It is easy for me to forget that the precarious state of my health affects not just me but also my friends, one of whom told me he felt sad that he might lose me. I was very touched. Yet he might not – at least not from the cancer. I'm in such a paradoxical position. I might be completely cured – or dead from the cancer in a year or two. If I am cured I am unlikely ever to know, but I will certainly know, eventually, if I am not. Damocles' sword will dangle above my head by an ever-fraying thread for my remaining days, but, should I look up, which most of us rarely do, would I see anything other than a harmless spider?

Yet there is a deeper paradox. Before cancer, I was happy. During diagnosis and treatment, I was no less so, and I remain so, despite the greater uncertainty of my life and the discomforts and inconveniences cancer has brought. Indeed, I am probably happier than I have ever been. I was teaching regularly again, having just begun a six-week introductory course on Buddhism and meditation. Nothing makes me happier than communicating the Dharma.

Falling leaves and failing legs

Then came another test – my legs were getting weaker, even though I had been neither swimming nor cycling for weeks, and despite walking much less than during the early weeks of my recovery. It was a conundrum.

I had been to Redditch, near Birmingham, to see my dentist, Jayabodhi, but the effort had cost me dear. Then for three days I had rested my legs, yet their strength seemed to be ebbing. What did they need – exercise or rest? I opted for the former and asked Gus to accompany me on a walk, lest I get stranded.

We reached the park, but I couldn't go much further, so we paused by the bridge over the canal and I eased my weight against the parapet, luxuriating in the mildness of this late November day. The light was all but horizontal, catching the lingering yellow on the trees, alchemizing it into purest gold: the most poignant moment in autumn – and my most precious – the last few leaves clinging with but the slightest grip to their life source, hanging on to face their fate – a gentle fall to earth, or a taunting flight heavenwards, that they might then be cast down like fallen angels, a choice not theirs to make.

'Here, look through these', Gus said, handing me his tinted shades, and the subtlest gold was transmuted into brilliant copper: spectacular, but gaudy, counter-alchemical.

*

I needed advice, and so I called a prostate cancer nurse. 'It's not just the radiotherapy that's caused the fatigue', she insisted. Chemo and hormone therapy were also culpable. The latter blocks the production of testosterone, which is important in helping to maintain muscle mass.

'The fatigue could continue as long as you are on leuprorelin', she warned. What a wonderful exercise in patience that might be! Fourteen more months, with possibly an additional twelve, on shivering shanks! 'But it could also clear up within two months. There's no predictable pattern', she added reassuringly.

'So what can I do?'

'Learn to manage it.' Is that not what I had been trying to do? 'It's a matter of trial and error.' But I had had many trials and had made as many errors. 'If you do too much one day, you will simply have less energy the next. You can't damage anything.' But it's a double bind: if I do too much, I fatigue my legs, and if I get insufficient weight-bearing exercise, such as walking, I will lose more muscle mass, which will compound the fatigue.

I rested for two more days until, at last, my insatiable appetite drove me to the park to savour again its autumnal beauty. Although the overnight gale had diminished, countless fallen leaves were yet restless on whatever beds they had found. The trees that had moved me so much a few days earlier were now bare, their glory surrendered, like reluctant Richard's crown, to an implacable force. By the time I returned to the LBC, I doubted my legs could keep me upright, they seemed so ready to give way.

And then the beast slunk heavily into my mind – Doubt. Will my energy return? Why had I been tricked by its revival then mocked by its wane? Will I permanently lose the use of my legs? Irrational, of course.

I reminded myself that my energy would recover by morning. But what if it did not? If this was just the beginning of a steady decline, what would I do? And would it really matter? I could still hear Mitsuko Uchida play Schubert, though perhaps not in concert as I hoped to do the following week. I would continue to write and would write more. I could still meet people and lead a fulfilling life – it would not stop me teaching.

The girl and the eagle

As these and similar thoughts drifted through my mind, my attention was drawn to a girl, of perhaps nine or ten, in school uniform. It was now dark and, during an idle moment, I watched her from our bathroom, two stories above the street, as she mimicked a pole dancer in the café opposite. She was dancing in a floor-length window – revealed and obscured by its broken condensation – empty tables and chairs extending behind her; her mother at one side, consumed by her food, oblivious to the dance. I was its sole spectator, touched by the girl's innocence, amused by her precocious talent, struck by this supposedly enticing routine robbed of its sensuality.

It might have been the following morning; I was in a ruined abbey on the edge of a major city when a large eagle landed on the remnants of a wall a few metres away. A distinctive white collar highlighted its dark brown plumage, the latter mismatched with its scuffed, and decidedly lighter-toned, shoes, several sizes too big for its feet. I'm a great lover of nature, but, frankly, it looked ridiculous. Had the shoes been of the right size and coordinated with its feathers, possibly I would have thought less harshly of its appearance, but, when it turned its diminutive anthropoid face to look at me, there was no chance.

Why had this regal creature been reduced to this absurdity, its penetrating eyes dead as buttons, its fearsome bill broken off, its offensive talons tamed... or had some hideous deformity displaced *them*? I stared back uncomprehendingly until I awakened.

It was the first dream I had remembered for a very long time. My sleep had been excessively fitful for months, so when I had at last sunk into the profoundest slumber this mockery on stolen wings had stolen in.

What goes down must come up

When I began cancer treatment, I had been relieved of community chores – washing up, cooking, and cleaning – everything. The men in my community were happy to do these things for me, and I was deeply grateful. Nonetheless, I still wanted to contribute. Consequently, I continued to buy our fruit thrice weekly from a nearby market stall, as it was relatively easy for me to do this with a trolley bag. On returning, I would leave the bag downstairs for others to bring up; sometimes, however, I would do so myself – perhaps unwisely.

One day, I was halfway up the stairs dragging a large bag of bananas, pushing myself up backwards with my arms, when one of my community members caught me. He paused, regarding this laughable sight with both concern and amusement.

'Where there's a will there's a way', he said drily, yet slightly accusingly (I thought), as if I was a recidivist apprehended in some nefarious activity yet again.

('Honest, Guv, I'd never do this in public. No! Not even on the Underground.' I know others find me eccentric, but I do retain *some* sense of dignity.) He kindly relieved me of my swag.

'I *can* actually climb the stairs', I said, somewhat weakly. 'I'm just trying to conserve my energy.' Was he convinced? More pertinently, was I?

I *must* do something about my legs. Niccala had recommended chi kung, and so I took it up again, together with a simple exercise for developing muscle mass. A week later my strength began to return, enabling me to hear Mitsuko play three sonatas by Schubert at the Festival Hall.

She strode briskly to the piano in her golden shoes, then, after a cursory bow, without pause, she struck the opening chords, which resounded dramatically around the hall. It was a golden evening, not because of her meticulously coordinated attire or the light that bathed her, nor yet her natural grace – nor even the humility that ennobles the truly gifted. The final piece (D850), played with a sublime touch, utterly transported me. Perhaps my sensibilities, heightened by recent experience, were elevated still further by music born of the imagination of one who – though yet young – knew he was fatally ill.

I felt grateful that I was not a musician, especially not a highly accomplished one like Mitsuko. Immersing myself day after day in such exalted music, as *she* does, might have deafened me to the song of impermanence now singing constantly in my ear.

Another man from the LBC had just died of prostate cancer – the second in three months. A few weeks earlier the cancer of an old friend, with the same diagnosis as mine, had recurred. I had been expecting to co-lead a four-year study course commencing in the new year, but this had been allocated to two other Order members lest I should die before completing it. But, most significantly, 25 December was just three weeks away. Should I awaken on Christmas Day, I would have lived longer than my father. I half expected not to do so.

Spinning

I sometimes feel as if consciousness is seeking a divorce from the body (on grounds, perhaps, of physical cruelty). It's a pleasing sensation, but probably it is simply a misperception of fatigue. My physical fatigue was obvious to anybody, but its mental counterpart still affected me, perhaps more than I cared to admit.

But maybe it is the other way around – that this body wants rid of its troublesome spirit – hence the mad spinning in my head, as if my whole body was in an ever more furious whirl like an Olympic athlete desperate to cast his hammer beyond silver.

And its slimy trick: the accompanying nausea – when it is that severe, you just want to die at once. My usual response was to pass out, leaving this body well behind – seemingly released into another universe – only to awaken in its vomit, as I had done on several occasions in India.

But there was a new carpet, and it spun at a pace well beyond my madly turning brain. It was a *new* carpet; I mustn't. I stood up, staggered towards the door, reeled through another, fumbled along a darkened corridor, slid against its wall, stumbled down steps, and hung my head over the bath – not in shame, but in relief.

Had I remembered, I would have had my bucket by me, but I had dispensed with it, thinking it would no longer be needed after I had finished radiotherapy (which I wrongly imagined had caused the dizziness). However, the dizzy spells had continued and gradually intensified for weeks after. Then I recalled that this dreadful swirling had overwhelmed my brain two years previously, before cancer had slipped surreptitiously into my life.

I had completely forgotten about benign paroxysmal positional vertigo. Surely, I could be forgiven; the name itself trips your tongue, spins your head, and forbids remembrance. Finally, I had recognized it, and again began the contorted exercises necessary to cure it.

*

'Your pulses are quite deficient', Niccala had said, and so the following week I asked her, 'Am I about to fall off my perch, do you think?'

'No, it's just the effect of the [cancer] treatments you've had. Your body needs time to recover.' She paused before adding, 'You do realize that this has aged you.'

Age had stared back at me from a mirror, months before, but she was the first to say it, and I was grateful. The final vestiges of my prime were being drawn from my blood, eroded from my face, and sapped from my limbs.

'I have a mirror', I said, but her words highlighted the

reality. No matter how youthful I might feel inwardly, my body was visibly decaying – paradox and conflict. The spirit trapped inside this physical wreck was in rebellion.

The following day, my legs were so weak I could again hardly walk. The culprit was not acupuncture, but a cold; for three days, at its height, I struggled up the thirty-seven stairs to my room, then a further treatment restored more vitality – but not for long.

Still, I had now completed the six-week Dharma course and a few days later I travelled, unaided, to Adhisthana for the LBC winter retreat.

Surely?

The following day, I met Bhante. We talked mostly about writing – his, mine, and that of Henry Miller, whom Bhante had been re-reading. He had read my cancer pieces and had found them funny yet horrific. Though I had exploited my humour, I had not intended to horrify and was startled at the thought that he and others experienced my words in this way.

Why had he returned to Miller, whose writing he considered to be of mixed quality? He cited, as an example, Miller's poignant account of a clergyman helping his father to deal with alcoholism. Discussing literature with Bhante brought back countless memories of the times we had lived together, but then a loud knock on the door told me it was time to go.

'I hope we'll meet again', I said, grasping his hand as I was about to leave.

'Surely, we will', he responded, smiling. Surely? How 'surely', I wondered, as conscious of *his* mortality as of mine.

I headed for the door, but then turned back. '*Hopefully*, not *surely*', I said. He had not heard, and so I repeated my words, increasing their volume. Now he understood and smiled, though I forget what he said. I never saw him again.

Two days later, I awakened, conscious that it was Christmas Day.

8

Surviving

Surviving cancer is as much about contending with the after-effects of radical treatment as it is about defeating the disease. Having been through chemo and radiotherapy, and still in the midst of hormone therapy, I was left with my physical vitality utterly depleted.

My energy would come and go as unpredictably as the wind, yet as surely as the ebbing and flowing of the tide. 'You'll be surprised at just how quickly your energy will return', one of my radiographers had assured me, but, to me, its return seemed uncertain. One man, recovering from the same treatments for prostate cancer, told me that his vitality had not revived.

At the end of the LBC winter retreat at Adhisthana, fifteen weeks after completing radiotherapy, I had such a dramatic lapse in strength that I could barely walk twenty metres, and it was difficult to resist the thought that perhaps my loss was permanent. Or could it simply be the continuing effects of leuprorelin, as one prostate-cancer nurse maintained?

It would have been impossible for me to travel home by train and Underground. Fortunately, a retreatant kindly drove me back in his spacious, new BMW, and so I returned to Sukhavati in style. On arrival, the driver and his friend virtually carried me upstairs – each with one hand grabbing the back of my trouser belt, their other hand gripping the stair rails. With my arms hanging over their shoulders, I laughed all the way, urging them to go ever faster.

A few days later, I shuffled into Niccala's acupuncture clinic greeted by her laughter. 'My energy has gone again', I explained unnecessarily.

'I'm not surprised. I'm impressed it lasted so long.'

*

Several times during the ensuing months, I gained then lost energy, but always with a slight overall increase, so it seemed. But my strength was ever fickle. I was frequently the victim of over-optimism, having to abandon one attempt to go to a concert at the Wigmore Hall and occasional efforts to reach Victoria Park. This never seriously hindered my teaching commitments, but, just a few minutes after giving the first of two talks in Oxford in February, I was exhausted, even though while I was speaking I had felt as vital as ever. Nonetheless, I knew that I was never quite at my best, as I still suffered mildly from chemo brain – as if I was thinking in slow motion.

Niccala had a nutritional solution for my deficient brain, generously giving me a bottle of organic flaxseed oil. At an acupuncture session a few weeks later, I was inadvertently trapped in her store room, which serves as a second exit from her clinic. Just as I phoned for help, she burst into the room, 'I'm so sorry! I forgot to unlock the door this morning.'

'Oh… I thought it was an initiative test to see if my brain medicine was working.' Despite my failed attempt to solve the riddle of the door, the grey matter did seem to be functioning more efficiently.

Three score and ten

A few weeks later it was my seventieth birthday, for which I had been given the perfect gift – an opportunity to rouse and gladden the hearts of the Dharma-night class at the LBC with a talk on Milarepa. Three days later, the birthdays of myself and Gus were celebrated in our community. As is the custom at Sukhavati, everyone rejoiced in our merits. I have never been more appreciated and was moved. Shortly afterwards, I treated Gus to a performance of Mahler's fifth symphony at the Festival Hall to celebrate his twenty-eighth.

*

Several of my friends had suggested that chi kung sessions with Master Lam might help me. And so I arranged to see him. Because I was incapacitated by cancer treatment I had to book 'healing' sessions, but how these differed from chi kung was unclear to me, as he still taught me chi kung, although I had to practise while sitting.

His premises in Lambeth were reminiscent of so many places I have visited in Singapore, with the same ambient Chinese music tinkling in the background, and I felt immediately at home. He scrutinized me very carefully then said, 'You nee' maw exercise.' This was novel.

'What about swimming?'

'Swimmin' no' exercise', he replied firmly. 'Swimmin' for fun.'

'Walking?'

'Walkin' exercise', he nodded approvingly. At the end of the session he took another long look at me before saying, 'You no' so bad… many people worse.' A man of few words; simpatico – I liked him.

*

The first of my biannual cancer reviews was due, but first came the blood test. On the way to the hospital, I encountered Niccala at Bethnal Green Tube. The train was crowded, and so I headed for a seat indicating priority for the old and frail. As my GP had recently startled me by brazenly describing me to my face as 'elderly', I claimed my privilege. 'Do you mind if I sit there?' I enquired of the young man, perhaps a little pugnaciously. He made way for me, regarding me suspiciously as if I had somehow duped him. Apparently, I am not your average old codger, whatever my doctor thinks. Niccala grinned at me.

'Devamitra, it isn't obvious that you should have that seat', she said, sotto voce.

'But I'm seventy now', I objected, almost indignantly.

'Yes, but you bring such energy to what you do, it confuses people.' Hmm… perhaps.

When I reached my destination, I struggled to my feet with a touch of thespian exaggeration, glanced at the sceptical young man – who looked yet more doubtfully at me – then walked briskly away.

Two days later, I was back at the hospital for my results. 'Your PSA level is down to 0', my oncologist said, beaming at me.

'Signifying what?'

'It means it's undetectable. Fifty per cent of our review patients hit 0. You have a better chance of a cure.'

'Then I have even more reason to be grateful to you', I responded. Besides, she's such a pleasant woman, one is grateful for her very existence.

A muscle had gone into spasm inside my lower back, which I had understood to be a side-effect of radiotherapy delivered to the pelvis – though not according to her. But it was a problem, as it was increasingly painful and I was about to leave for a four-week solitary retreat at Guhyaloka, our isolated retreat centre hidden in the mountains close to Benidorm, in Spain.

*

Despite the pain, the following day, I queued two hours one morning for two 'day tickets' for *The Ferryman*. Perhaps that was unwise, but Jez Butterworth's play had left such a strong impression on me that I felt impelled to see it a second time, and this would be my last opportunity. Besides, I wanted both to test my resources and to treat Prajnamanas, whose birthday I would miss while I was away.

I enjoyed the play as much on the second occasion as I had

on the first, but, once in solitude a few days later, it frequently came to mind, raising the spectre of my Irish grandfather, his premature death, and his involvement in the IRA.

Solitude

The day before my departure for Guhyaloka, the pain in my pelvis was so severe that I thought seriously of cancelling, but, as I had an acupuncture appointment, I decided to wait and see if Niccala could fix it. Unfortunately, she failed. 'There is one last thing we can try', she assured me. 'Come back this evening. It'll only take a few minutes.'

Not thinking to ask what, I returned shortly before giving my second talk on Milarepa to the LBC Dharma-night class.

Bloodletting. Had she mentioned it earlier, I may have declined, but now that I was back – and feeling desperate – I submitted. A trickle of blood was released from a small vein in the back of my right leg and by the time I left the clinic the pain in my lower back was diminishing. By morning my back felt almost normal for the first time in two weeks. The improvement was extraordinary, and I travelled to Guhyaloka almost pain-free.

I had very reluctantly cancelled my retreat the previous year when undergoing chemotherapy. I had been deluded enough to think that I could manage both chemo and solitude at Guhyaloka, but the second round of chemo had finally dismissed that folly.

I was so happy to be back in the valley and to be once more in the hut where I had spent nine months in solitary retreat just four years previously, but I realized on my first day that it would be difficult. I was enervated and the pain in my pelvis was already returning and increasing – both probably consequences of the travel, I thought; surely, I would feel better by morning. But the following day the pain was worse and I was yet weaker. It was my most significant lapse in energy since the winter retreat. Had I come a month earlier, it would have been much easier, but now I wondered if I could continue and began to think I should not have come. Indeed, suddenly I did not want to be there. I was rapidly drifting towards despondency, but then realized what was happening.

I recognized the initial stages of a pattern that I had encountered several times before in solitude: resistance and reaction. I must be firm and get things in perspective. I did not wish to give way to weakness; and so, I reflected. This retreat, like others before, would present a unique challenge – probably the toughest I had yet faced. Once more I must embrace it and capitalize on it. Having resolved to do so, I felt the reaction subside and I was content. I awoke the following morning feeling completely happy with no desire to be anywhere else.

After meditating, I took my breakfast in my favourite spot, slightly to the side of the hut, beside a pine surrounded by rosemary and rock rose, amidst countless bees thirsting for their nectar. I have spent untold hours enjoying the view from this spot in spring, summer, autumn, and winter, yet have never tired of it.

The wind's bitter blast countered the warmth of the rising sun on my back, as I looked down from the edge of the crumbling terrace into the forest below and across to the mountains beyond.

Perhaps it was then, as I watched the birds flitting to and fro, that the thought drifted through my mind, 'This body is an old man.' It was oddly impersonal and strangely detached – not my thought, not my body.

Fear no more the heat o' th' sun,
Nor the furious winter's rages.[7]

Shakespeare's famous song was not in my mind at the time, though it might have been. What was the use of this body without its vitality? Had I known that cancer treatment would reduce me to this, I might have declined it. Such thoughts had been milling around in the back of my mind for a while and had surfaced strongly the previous evening. I had been forced yet again to ask myself, 'What is the point in continuing to live?' and I found the same answer as before – the only answer that gives my life meaning: that I have experience that others value and I feel a duty to preserve it for them.

Long after I had finished my breakfast, I continued to sit in company with the bees, in harmony with their song, feeling glad to be alive and fortunate to be in this place – despite everything. Gus, Prajnamanas, and other young friends came to mind and, as I relaxed further, a wave of gratitude welled up within, utterly transporting me.

*

But I knew I would have to conserve my energy; I had little to spare. As recommended by Master Lam, I practised chi kung thrice daily, as this always vitalized me. If I walked to and from the end of the track leading to my hut six times after each session of chi kung, I would complete the 10,000 steps I hoped to manage each day. That would help to keep my back mobile and perhaps resolve the spasm in my pelvis.

Notwithstanding my physical weakness, I was sorely tempted by a pile of logs awaiting their doom; chopping wood is so satisfying, but I could barely wield the axe. Given all my daily chores, that would have taxed me far too much. It was difficult enough just looking after myself. But I could not resist and took a swipe at a beckoning log, which gratifyingly split cleanly at the first blow. I was left breathless and my quivering legs threatened to give way, but it was wonderful, so I rationed myself to one log a day. The rest of the time I must be content just to sit and do nothing – and I was, deeply so.

Unlike previous years, I was unaffected by the shifting moods of the day. For many years, the onset of evening had always unsettled me in solitude, leaving me slightly melancholic and wanting company. I had often distracted myself from this unwanted sensation by going for a walk, but on my previous retreat I had realized that this mood was a natural, almost impersonal response to the shifting light. I had learned to relax into it and enjoy it. But now I felt perfectly content whatever the time of day, and could appreciate the constant, subtle changes in atmosphere.

Defeat

And so my retreat wore on with occasional unexpected encounters. I disturbed a large, brilliant green lizard in my washing-up bowl, sipping treasured drips from my rainwater tank. After a desperate scrabble on treacherous plastic, it swiftly scurried away on more certain terrain and disappeared into the log pile. Had I known he was there, I would have kept my distance, enjoyed his magnificence, and let him drink in peace. As I sat absorbed in the twilight one evening, a pine marten passed beneath my window, paused to bid me goodnight, then vanished before I could return his greeting.

I was perfectly content, despite the nagging pain in my back and the weakness of my legs, but after eleven days there was a dramatic change. I felt even weaker. I assumed that this was just another blip in my inconstant energy levels. I could barely stay awake in meditation, then dozed constantly as I sat in the early morning sun. The energy seemed to be draining out of my body, as if it was slowly drifting into the beyond and dragging me with it. I even dropped off during chi kung in the afternoon and, when I tried to walk afterwards, I reached the end of the track but struggled with every one of the hundred-odd steps back.

I sat down on my bed, rested, then decided to make some tea. The kettle had a swivel handle that was prone to falling to either side, as it did on this occasion. When the water had boiled, the handle was very hot, and so I used a small tea towel to grasp it. Unfortunately, the towel was made of synthetic material, which adhered to the side of the kettle. Not realizing that I could not get a proper grip on the handle, I almost spilled the water over myself.

Shaken, I sat on my bed again. I had had a similar incident with a pan of boiling soya milk the day before. Twice I had been lucky, but I could not afford to risk a third incident, and I realized that I was no longer capable of looking after myself. I even lacked sufficient energy to prepare my evening meal. Pondering this, I burst into tears and wept uncontrollably. I felt defeated; more seriously, the thought that an era of my life might finally have come to an end distressed me.

I had first come to Guhyaloka in September 1986, shortly after Subhuti had acquired the land. I had gone to lead study for the building team for a few weeks while Subhuti was away. I began going to Guhyaloka for solitary retreats shortly after the first hut had been completed. It was so wild and beautiful I never seriously considered going anywhere else and had returned at least for a month most years. The hut in which I was staying is spartan by Triratna standards – a bed, table and chair, woodstove, shrine, two gas rings for cooking, and a drop toilet a short distance from the hut. And the great blessing (and inconvenience) of no electricity. (Though, shortly after I left, a solar panel was installed – doubtless an improvement, but I felt a deep regret at this attenuation of simplicity.)

*

Very reluctantly I called the community and left a message asking for help. Half an hour later, a community member came and talked to me, and shortly afterwards I was driven down to the community bungalow where I spent the following three days before returning to London.

Shifting gates

Even were I disencumbered of luggage, the journey back would have been challenging. I could not walk very far, and the pain in my back was intensifying; I was further blessed with an involuntary limp. Neil, one of the community members, kindly volunteered to drive me to the airport and thoughtfully even took my bags as far as security. But then I was on my own.

I managed to get to the gate for my flight, but then the gate was changed, which called on more of my diminishing physical strength. The gods were evidently favouring me, testing my grit. Arriving at the second gate, I sat down with considerable satisfaction only to discover that the capricious gate number had changed again. By sheer force of will, I reached the third gate and finally boarded the plane.

After close on three hours of sitting, my limbs seemed to seize, rendering any movement of my right leg intolerably painful, and so I requested assistance from a flight attendant. Despite suffering the indignity of being wheelchaired off the plane, I was profoundly grateful.

I was parked with a number of others in a corridor to

wait for a buggy that would take us to the terminal entrance. Buggies came and went, but none of them would pick us up, which was a source of much griping and groaning among my fellow invalids, while I quietly enjoyed watching the planes come and go, confident that sooner or later we would get away.

Prajnamanas had texted me, asking whether or not he should arrange a taxi for me on arrival, but I had not replied. It was a generous offer from my friends, but the extravagance of a taxi from Gatwick to Bethnal Green was insupportable to my frugal mind. However, that was not the only consideration.

Kindness to oneself?

Years ago, when I was living at a retreat centre in Norfolk, some members of the community were unhappy about having to live in caravans. This had prompted Bhante to observe more generally that, if we were serious about practising the Dharma, we needed to toughen up. He even suggested that perhaps every Order member should spend six months working in India as part of their Dharma training. I took his comments to heart. Notwithstanding the importance of having a positive self-regard – so vital to one's psychological health – this is just one reason why I have always found the idea, so frequently voiced, of 'being kind to oneself' unappealing. It is so difficult to overcome my deep-rooted selfishness, I prefer to think of kindness as a way of reaching out to others and forgetting myself in a positive way.

It is certainly necessary to take care of oneself, which was why I left my retreat. In the circumstances that was probably objective – other members of my community seemed to think so – but it is so tempting to choose the softer options in life rather than meet its tougher challenges and overcome them. In leaving my retreat, had I merely given way to weakness?

The short distance from the terminal entrance to the train station seemed interminable on my failing limbs, but I knew that once I was on the train things would get easier. I was met at City Thameslink station and relieved of my luggage, and returned to the LBC on a number eight bus. I was both saddened and pleased to be back.

Later, I explained to Maitreyabandhu why I had returned. He looked at me knowingly. 'I'm not surprised', he said.

'No', I conceded, 'but unless you reach for the stars, you'll never travel far.'

*

I had been very unlucky. I had not just had an energy lapse; for the first time in my life, I had been suffering from sciatica – as I discovered when I saw Niccala, the day after my return.

A month later, my mind was again returning to Guhyaloka. I *must* go again! My energy was already reviving and the sciatica had gone, and so I booked another solitary retreat for the following year. Come what may, I would find a way to persevere.

9

Testosterone Toll

'They're just waiting for the cancer to recur', Niccala explained while treating me with acupuncture five months later, days before my next biannual review. That hadn't occurred to me. The gap between consultations means that you can forget about the cancer for another half year – except you never quite do. 'Scanxiety' is a term coined by cancer patients to describe the seemingly universal fear that increases the closer they get to their next scan. It doesn't trouble me, but, as the next review looms, my awareness of the precarious nature of my life intensifies. Once more, I am roused from complacency – so difficult to resist – and inevitably I wonder what news awaits me.

Double zero

'Your PSA level is at 0', the registrar informed me.

'Again?'

'Yes.'

'That's twice in succession.'

'As things stand, it's looking like you *might* be cured', she continued, cautiously. I couldn't respond to this; it was so unexpected. The possibility of a cure had seemed a distant, perhaps unlikely, prospect. I had become reconciled to life with cancer, assuming that it would eventually kill me, but this siren song had reduced me to silent incredulity; then there was a knock on the door.

'Ah, there you are!' said my consultant, stepping into the room. 'I was just on my way to collect you… Like the hair', she said, commenting on my lengthening, grey locks. Most fitting; by prescribing chemotherapy, she had been principally responsible for the loss of their predecessors.

'And *you've* turned black', I responded referring to the startling colour of her hair.

'That's very observant of you', she remarked, evidently pleased; 'most men don't even notice.'

'I've hit 0 again', I said, now that we'd exchanged pleasantries.

'I noticed. That's very good news.' I was beginning to take it in.

After she'd gone, I asked the registrar, 'Can I come off the hormone therapy?' She need not have answered; her guarded expression told me all.

'We generally recommend three years for high-risk patients.' Seemingly, there is still a high risk that my cancer will spread. I was too slow to see the apparent inconsistency at the time. 'We're still waiting for the results of the latest studies', she responded, after I had asked – results that could mean that my term might be reduced from three to two years. 'We'll let your GP know immediately if you can stop.' But I heard nothing further, and understood that there was to be no respite.

It changes nothing. Unless I am told unequivocally that I am cured, I would rather not hear the word spoken. But it would have been pleasant to have been acquitted from the seemingly endless cycle of boom and bust with my physical energy, should leuprorelin prove to be its cause.

*

I left the hospital disoriented, wishing the registrar's conditional words had never been spoken, as they seemed to have me almost in thrall. Returning from the consultation, I met Matt, a young saxophonist, on his way to a rehearsal, and told him what she had said. Although I stressed the qualifications with which she had protected the final word, his face lit up, clearly delighted. How could it not? But I felt uneasy, as if I had tempted fate by revealing a secret that should have been buried in my mind, and yet so quickly I had revealed it for all to hear.

This was not mere superstition. I could not quite believe her words, and sought to shed their complacency-inducing influence. Trying to forget them or force them out of my mind was counterproductive.

The only way forward was to see their vanity – to note each qualifying phrase and word, aware of its unreliability. 'As things stand…' But things never stand; they constantly shift and change, bewilderingly, capriciously so – frequently defying logic and expectation. 'It's looking like…' Ah, but things often 'look like' only to deceive and disappoint. 'You *might* be…' *Might!* 'Might' is a whole universe of possibilities that can turn on you with contradictions, flouting the hopes it inspires. It is not that I seek certainties, but I do not seek hopes. Such innocent, well-intentioned words cannot but tempt the Furies to taunt an unguarded mind when linked finally with the most seductive word in a cancer patient's vocabulary. I must be vigilant.

It was strange, even perverse, but, now that the immediate threat to my life had seemingly receded, I almost regretted the change. For all the terrible discomforts of chemo and radiotherapy, and their uncertain outcome, they had been accompanied by heightened awareness and an underlying exhilaration. My life had seemed a thing of gossamer at the mercy of shifting winds – as, actually, it always is – but I was constantly reminded of that, and, though at times I forgot, I could not do so for long.

Moreover, my mind had relaxed quite profoundly, as if there was nothing to cling to anymore. I had had little choice, because often I was so incapacitated by my treatments that all I could do was surrender to their effects – even try to enjoy them. Simply looking out of the window of my room, listening to the most sublime music, unable to do anything else, had quite transported me at times. But then it all faded, like a forgotten dream.

Coffee?

Winter was almost upon us. For several months my energy had been building. I had not felt so physically vital since commencing chemo, then suddenly I had another relapse, albeit less severe than previously. On one occasion when Niccala was away, Andrew, one of her acupuncture colleagues, treated me. He examined my legs and assured me that they felt strong, not weak, and that the problem was caused by toxic overload. I needed to detox. Niccala agreed.

The discomfort came to a head when I began experiencing an unpleasant tingling for several hours after showering, which often kept me awake at night. This had happened many times previously after swimming. My body seemed to be reacting to the water or something in it – perhaps chlorine. I had taken breaks from swimming, but I could hardly stop showering. Even just minimizing the contact between my body and the water did not prevent the tingling.

Niccala had been suggesting for some time that I use coffee enemas, but I was not keen. Eventually, I bought the necessary kit and even the special coffee, but I could not bring myself to use it. Although I am open to the idea of 'detoxing', I am aware that medical practitioners are generally dismissive of it. But it was not just my body that was troubling me.

*

Matt had asked me and another actor to read four poems by Thomas Hardy at an evening of jazz and poetry at The Gallery Café in Bethnal Green. He and four of his friends, all recently graduated from the Guildhall School, would provide the music. I had rehearsed long and hard, as I always do, and could probably have recited the poetry without the text before me, but I was increasingly mistrustful of my short-term memory.

My mental lapses were also affecting my teaching and my communication with others more and more. On the evening before my third biannual review, I was teaching at the LBC. I had prepared thoroughly and knew exactly what I wanted to say, but when the time came to speak I was unable to marshal my thoughts properly; my coherency had morphed into a tangle, so it seemed to me.

At the heart of my diminishing mental acuity was a compound of progressively severe short-term memory loss, slowness of mind, and occasional cognitive confusion. I had tried to communicate this to the registrar at my previous consultation, but it was a subtle matter difficult for me to articulate and she had not properly understood. Six months later, however, it was more pronounced.

More erections

Spring had sprung, seemingly early, with the promise of vigorous renewal. My energy, in sync with the sap, was rising, and I was back at the hospital.

As I approached her consulting room, I noticed my oncologist had a rather callow-looking youth sitting by her, and so I hesitated before entering.

'Do come in', she said, welcoming me, bright and breezy and as friendly as ever. 'I haven't seen you for a long time.'

'No, indeed.'

'You don't mind having a medical student present?' I glanced at the bespectacled youth, who, had she not told me otherwise, could have been a truant.

'No. I always enjoy an audience.' I sat beside her desk; she immediately began her questions and I submitted to her scrutiny.

'How are you?'

'Very well, really', I replied somewhat slowly, trying to shake off my mental fatigue, as I met her lively eyes.

'Your PSA is still at 0', mentioning it as if it was now only to be expected. No reference to a cure; I was oddly relieved.

'A hat-trick... right... well, I suppose that's it then', I said stumbling over my words, expecting to be dismissed, and forgetting about the routine questions that she then rapidly fired at me. I felt like an actor constantly slow on cue in a pacey dialogue. Why was I so slow this morning?

'Bowels okay?'

'Yes.'

'Waterworks?'

'Fine.'

'Erections?' This was a topic she had never raised with me before, though several of her colleagues had. The question was slipped in so deftly, like a striker sending a goalkeeper the wrong way, I was momentarily nonplussed. I will probably never get used to being asked this so disinterestedly by a woman whose eyes simultaneously search mine for the truth. I'd better not fib.

'Rarely', I said, uncertain whether or not I still had them. Actually, I don't – not that they were particularly plentiful before I started treatment.

'Would you like some help with that?' What can a man say? Such genuine concern in a fellow's failing equipment – though clinical – is truly touching. Of course, she has to ask. Some men might be too embarrassed to raise it.

'No! I'm seventy-one now', I explained limply.

'Oh, age doesn't matter.' Perhaps she was not convinced. It must be rare to encounter a man genuinely uninterested in revitalizing his flaccid token of manhood.

'Really… I'm not bothered.'

I don't even think about such matters so vitally important to the young; had I been several decades younger… But even then, in my priapic youth, that intumescent piece of flesh could be a thorough nuisance, constantly bulging behind my flies, almost peeping above my belt – and *so* uncomfortable – me forever praying that it might subside, anxious lest someone notice. Life is so much easier without all that. Besides, virility is considerably more than the mere capacity for glorious and sustainable erections.

I must have finally convinced her. 'He is not concerned regarding erections', stated the letter to my GP summarizing our consultation, a copy of which I received a week or two later. This extraordinary fact was communicated twice in the course of its brief summary for the benefit of the various doctors, mostly female, who work at my local surgery; hopefully that will stifle any incredulity that might emanate from that quarter, so that my phallus can rest in peace for another six months.

'Anything else?' continued my oncologist.

'I still have a lot of fatigue in my legs. I suppose that's the hormone therapy.'

'Yes. The plan is to keep you on it until 2020.' Not that I expected otherwise. Still, it had only nine more months to run and then my fatigue should diminish.

*

I left the hospital having forgotten to mention my sluggish mind – which was symptomatic of the problem. Consequently, I decided to call the Prostate Cancer UK helpline – a ticklish business as there is no telling where such an innocent topic might lead.

When enquiring about the fatigue in my legs a few months previously, I had foolishly thought myself on safe ground, but the favoured topic had arisen at once. 'When you start getting erections again, you will know that the effects of leuprorelin are beginning to recede', I was told.

However, this time I was prepared. I recounted my problem to the nurse taking my call. 'It's very common', she assured me. 'Many men suffer from poor concentration. Part of the problem is that there are certain receptors in the brain that need testosterone to activate them, and there is no testosterone in your body', she explained. 'It will take a while, after treatment is ended, for your mental capacities to return to normal', she warned me. It was a relief to know that it was not degenerative.

'Weeks, months, years?'

'Several months… up to a year… maybe two. It varies a lot… Hormone therapy thrusts you into a premature old age', she added. This much I already understood. 'How old are you?'

'Seventy-one.'

'Oh, you don't sound it!' That, at least, was gratifying.

Sweating it out

Meanwhile, I had been looking further into 'detoxifying'. As perspiration is regarded as a detoxifying process, the obvious thing to do was to go to a sauna. With some difficulty I had managed to find an affordable sauna at a nearby leisure centre. When I arrived to book my third session, it was very busy and so I had to wait for fifty minutes. I approached the middle-aged woman with bottle-blond hair and startlingly red lips sitting at the membership desk. 'When is the quietest time to come?' I asked her.

'Oh, they can't come next week; it'll be empty.' I had no idea to whom she was referring.

'Right… well, actually I'm booked in for today, but generally when is it quieter?'

'Well, they're all coming today coz they can't come next week. So, like I said it won't be a problem next week.' My testosterone-starved brain was struggling. 'The 'ole place'll be empty including the pool and the gym', she continued.

'It's really nice', she added with an encouraging smile.

'Good… I'll certainly come, but what's the best time to avoid having to wait?'

'Any time you like, because they won't be here.' She must have thought me thoroughly thick. Perhaps my jaw had dropped. We really were not getting through to each other.

'So, why won't they be here?' I asked, tentatively, still wondering who 'they' might be.

'Coz there's some things they can't do in Ramadan.' Now I understood. She gave me the dates. What a pity; Ramadan mostly coincided with my solitary retreat.

'So, when Ramadan's finished, what are the quiet times?'

'Oh, come in June. They won't be 'ere then neeva coz they go on their 'olliedays to Bangladesh.'

'Good…' But truly I was perplexed; I gave it one last go. 'Are there *any* times that are *generally* quiet, when I can come?'

'Peak times.'

'Peak times are *quiet*?'

'Yeah, it's empty.' Evidently, I really was dense and so she helped me further in a slightly confidential tone. 'Nobody comes, coz they don't want to pay four pounds sixty for their sowna.' How tempting. I could have the whole place to myself at the 'busiest' time. But I didn't; there were plenty of people willing to pay that amount.

Once inside the sauna, during a brief hiatus in the Qawwali, I asked, 'Are you not permitted to take a sauna during Ramadan?'

'We are permitted, but it is not advised', explained my affable middle-aged neighbour. It is not difficult to understand why.

'You're getting old...'

A week or so later, I left for my annual solitary retreat in the Spanish mountains, which, unlike the previous year, went smoothly – despite a recurrence of severe sciatica and yet another lapse of energy. Oh, and yes, of course, I did break a tooth on an olive stone! But, in the past year, I had learned how to treat the sciatica, and, although it disrupted my retreat, it did not prevent me from doing what I had to do.

I stayed for the full four weeks, enjoying the bliss of solitude in company with the animals. While I was breakfasting one morning, with my legs stretched out before me, my feet resting on a convenient rock, a large, mostly silver lizard emerged from the undergrowth and stood at my feet for a minute or more, seemingly studying me closely, before slowly taking his leave. Such close contact with nature refreshes my spirit and always evokes a sense of awe – and even of tenderness for living things. Catching the ibex unawares, downwind from their sensitive nostrils, savouring their majesty for a few precious moments until a chance noise disturbs their quiet grazing, is utterly thrilling.

As one gets older, solitude becomes more and more challenging. Though I find it hard to say, or even believe, at least for the moment, I have become a bit frail. Consequently, Maniraja, anxious for my well-being, had discussed various scenarios with other members of the Guhyaloka community should things go wrong.

A few years previously, when I was a mere stripling of sixty-five, he had wanted to brief me before I disappeared into nine months of solitude inside the same hut. He was clearly struggling to raise the delicate matter troubling him, and I had had to prompt him. 'You're getting old, Devamitra', he had reminded me, quite unnecessarily, looking at me pointedly, with all the assurance of a man almost twenty years younger.

'You mean, what if I die?'

'Well… yes.'

'But I don't intend to die', I had quipped, facetiously.

I am incapable of resisting solitude, which I have learned to love. Although I am untroubled by the thought of dying alone, I would not wish my death to be a burden to those catering to my needs from a distance in such a remote place; I sympathized with Maniraja's concern.

Because of my age, I am increasingly susceptible of being rendered incapable by some acute medical occurrence, but that is a risk I am willing to take. Besides, even now, the chances of this happening are relatively low. My whole life has been a preparation – a training – for my final years, a gradual tendency towards increased fortitude in the face of adversity. I am indebted to my cancer for having brought me to the brink so many times – though I struggle to remain there; without cancer, perhaps I could not have sustained such an attitude with equanimity. Rarely do I experience flashes of anxiety, but, should they arise, I do not indulge them and they disappear from whence they came. Cancer has strengthened my resolve.

I left my retreat deeply satisfied, having managed to engage more with meditation than had been possible in recent years due to chronic back pain. I was sorry to be leaving, but I would be back. I still hungered for another relatively long solitary retreat of six months or more. I hoped I would not have to wait until my next life before satisfying my appetite.

Maniraja drove me out of the valley down to Benidorm bus station for the airport bus. 'See you next year' was my perennial valediction, heedless of the many assumptions hiding behind so few words. It was the last time I saw his cheery face. Within weeks, he was found collapsed in a chair in his hut, and I was forcibly struck by the ironies of both life and death.

... yet still you fall in love

Just minutes before embarking on my flight back to London, I realized I had lost my phone. I could not go back through the gate, so, on entering the cabin, I requested the attractive young black woman overseeing boarding to ask the ground staff if they could find it. She noted my seat number and the details of my phone. 'I'll see what I can do and, if it turns up before we leave, I'll bring it to you', she said. Immediately, she halted the boarding, stepped onto the bridge, and spoke to someone on my behalf before resuming her task.

This must have been one of the busiest moments in her day; perhaps she was simply following company guidelines, yet without the least hint of irritation she acted so graciously and efficiently, I was both touched and impressed. I would have forgiven her had she said, 'I'm sorry, but it's too late; can't you see how busy I am?' But she didn't. I took my seat, resigning myself to the likelihood that my phone was gone.

As she closed the door and continued to prepare the flight for departure, I forgot about my phone, and began to read. A few minutes later I glanced up to see her striding briskly down the aisle. 'Your phone, sir', she said, simultaneously thrusting it into my hand and then, without pause, returning to the bulkhead to demonstrate the safety procedures. Before I realized what had happened, she was gone and I had had no time to thank her. I was not content to leave it at that.

Later, well into the flight, when she was casually talking with her colleagues, I caught her attention and thanked her. She seemed rather taken aback. 'You got my phone back', I explained. 'You've saved me a lot of inconvenience.'

Her face lit up in recollection, then, with a smile whose radiant warmth was guaranteed to sear an old man's susceptible heart, she said, 'Oh, we always try to help people, sir!' An hour or so later, as I was about to disembark, she smiled again, asking, rather mischievously, 'Still got your phone, sir?'

'You bet', I replied, as I turned to go with a spring in my step that surprised me, perhaps a little in love, and certainly grateful. Such a small act of kindness had put a golden glow on the rest of my day. If I was in love, it was not just with her but with the entire universe.

Bust again

It had taken me a long time to realize that I had seriously underestimated the considerable fatigue, both mental and physical, I had suffered from leuprorelin. But more recently I had noticed a shift. My cycles of boom and bust had changed. My lapses were progressively less severe, my recovery quicker; slowly, slowly, I was feeling more vital. I could walk faster and sustain my speed for longer. I could stand for minutes on end without having to sit down. I could even meditate more frequently without falling asleep, and I was less prone to mental lapses. Nonetheless, fatigue still dogged me, catching me unawares.

Summer had carelessly cast the last remnants of its warmth to the bitter contempt of easterly and northerly winds; autumn chill had caught the air. It was late October. As had become my habit, I rose early, had breakfast, and left the community for the hospital while no one else was around. I did not wish to be seen leaving, lest anyone should ask where I was going. First the blood test then, two days later, the consultation. I preferred to let the others know after the latter, always on a Thursday, thus coinciding with our community night. Should my cancer recur, I could inform everyone together and spare myself the trouble of repeated conversations – hence my uncharacteristic clandestine behaviour.

As I left to brave the early morning Underground crush, I felt that something was not right, but I knew not what. It was cold, damp, and uncommonly dark. I had often descended through thousands of feet of unbroken cloud when flying into Heathrow; perhaps even now, five miles of dense vapour was suspended above my head, yearning for release. Or could some malevolent spirit have trapped the city beneath its oppressive mantle, depriving it of life-giving light and stifling my habitual buoyancy?

I had the first appointment of the day, but already clinical oncology was running twenty minutes late; by late morning, the delay could be much longer, which was why I always tried to get in first. During the past three years I had spent many hours waiting in this fluorescent place, its busy corridors resounding with countless footsteps, subdued voices, and the mournful tone of an electronic bell summoning its patients to good news or bad. Cancer on one side, heart on the other, and, in between, a huge void rising several floors, the chemo ward at the very top, radiotherapy buried in the basement in a confusion of yet more, seemingly endless, corridors.

Bell...
I kept glancing at the appointment screen, waiting for my name to flash up to the accompaniment of that awful sound; when, finally, it did, I walked briskly down the corridor to the consulting rooms, as if in flight from the bell's discordant notes echoing in the void. Perhaps Donne lurked somewhere

in the recesses of my mind, insisting that the bell tolled for me, that it always had, and that it always would. Or maybe, four centuries after his famous meditation,[8] his spirit still haunted the ghost of the burned-out cathedral, once close by. But that bell, that taunting bell, penetrated the core of my being, unfailingly this morning.

I knew exactly where I was going – turn left at the end, where her door would be ajar in discreet welcome, so characteristic of the woman. 'You're quick', my oncologist remarked, slightly taken aback, as I entered. 'Most patients take a while to get here... My system hasn't fully loaded yet', she continued, her attention split between me and her computer screen. As always, unlike many of her female medical colleagues, she was meticulously turned out, on this occasion in a pink dress. It was a relief to be once more in natural light, and it was always a pleasure to meet her.

'I don't hang around', I responded, smiling at her by way of greeting. Neither did she.

'Your PSA is still at 0.' She paused for a moment. 'When is your final hormone injection?'

'Later today.' After a moment I asked tentatively, 'Do I really need it?' She pondered a moment before looking at me.

'To be honest, I don't know. We do know that men with your diagnosis need more than two years, but whether that's two and a half, or three years, is uncertain.'

I appreciated her candour, and was grateful for the space to consider. After a few moments of reflection, I responded resignedly, 'Okay… I'll go ahead.' Having come this far, why miss the final shot of the thirteen?

'That'll take you through to January.'

'So presumably my PSA will start to rise again after that.'

'Yes, but, provided it does not go above 2, I will not be concerned… If it does, I will have to ask for further tests', she said with a warning look, whose effect pierced the pit of my stomach, which, primed by the bell, now opened to an infinite abyss; back to reality. The deeper lessons of life and death are so hard to learn. Often, I think I have finally understood them, when I have merely forgotten. Worse still, no matter how constantly the messengers of death issue reminders, I wilfully ignore them until caught unawares, as on this occasion. Because my results had been consistently good, it had been tempting to think that maybe I was getting clear. Though I had vigorously resisted such thoughts, perhaps I had been unconsciously seduced by the registrar's incautious words, twelve months before.

'I'm still quite fatigued, presumably from the hormone therapy', I responded, having registered her glance, unable to resist raising this matter yet again.

'The chemo and radiotherapy as well', she chipped in; 'you have been subjected to very severe treatments.' That would explain the steady overall improvement I had sensed.

'So when can I expect my energy to return to normal?'

'Maybe another fifteen months.'

... and bones

A second DEXA scan, which the oncologist had arranged after our previous meeting, revealed a slight worsening of the bone density in my spine. 'That's almost certainly due to hormone therapy', she explained.

'So I have osteoporosis?'

'Yes, but marginally.' She offered me the standard treatment, but I declined.

'Are there any other long-term side effects?'

'An increased risk of cardiovascular disease, but it's marginal… and it's not clear from the study whether or not that's a consequence of hormone therapy; most men who get prostate cancer smoke, drink, are overweight, and don't exercise.' None of these conditions applied to me, as she knew very well, which once more begged the question, 'why did *I* get it?' How pointless even to ask. I will never know why – and neither will she.

*

I strode rapidly away from the hospital in the torrential rain now descending on the city, only to be checked by my leaden muscles, reducing my pace to what seemed like a crawl. Now I understood what was wrong. The station seemed further and further away as I became progressively wetter and colder, my vitality slowly sapping into the ground. The coincidence between the weather, my strange mood, that warning glance, and yet another lapse, all on the very day of my final dose of leuprorelin, caused me to reflect. So many strands were perhaps woven together – biochemical, seasonal, psychosomatic, past mental habits, and perhaps even a state of consciousness beyond the mundane.

An hour or so later, I attended a meeting about one of the classes at the LBC, but I might just as well not have been there. My mind was once more sluggish, incoherent, even tenebrous, as if I was half blind, struggling to identify shifting objects, now revealed, then obscured in a swirling mist.

I left early for another soaking in the incessant rain for that final injection marking the beginning of the end of three years of cancer treatment. My spirits should have been high, but they were as low as the saturated cloud base above – but even such a brooding sky could not hold them down for long. By evening, my natural buoyancy had soared well beyond the influence of that vaporous mass and I was thankful to be alive. I was confident that this latest dip in energy, relatively severe though it was, would not last, and within a week I was once more on the upward spiral; by the new year, my physical vitality was almost back to normal.

Epilogue

More blood

'Which would you recommend?', I asked the GP. She had suggested two options after examining me.

'The colonoscopy', she replied, firmly, but kindly. 'Had you been under fifty, I would not refer you; it's because of your age', she assured me, sensing my reluctance. 'I'm pretty sure that it's just a haemorrhoid that we can't see. I'm only referring you because of the guidelines.'

'Could it not be a side effect of radiotherapy?'

'Extremely unlikely; it's well over two years since you had it.'

There had been more blood, this time not from my penis, but from its near neighbour. It had happened several times during the preceding weeks. 'It would be rotten luck to get two cancers in a row', I said, philosophically.

'It happens; one cancer does not give you immunity to others.' I knew that; it had happened to the sister of a friend. And surely it could not be caused by a metastasis of my prostate cancer; only six weeks earlier my PSA level was still at 0.

'I was hoping to avoid a colonoscopy', I confessed, almost wearily. 'I've had two gastroscopies in the past.'

'Oh, they are worse!' She glanced at her computer screen, presumably at my file. 'Where did you have them?'

'The first was in India…'

'In *India*?', she asked incredulously, perhaps a little horrified, as she turned back to face me.

'Yeah… without sedation.' What a fraud! There had been nothing heroic in that; I had had no choice.

*

I dragged my feet to the hospital for the consultation, as the possibility of more cancer treatment was more than I could stomach. I had regretted agreeing to the colonoscopy and played down my symptoms when interviewed by the African nurse; but she was tough and not to be hood-winked.

'We need to know where that blood is coming from', she insisted as we eyeballed one another. I submitted by silent consent… Or was I merely being wimpish in the presence of this formidable woman?

'You can only eat foods on this list for forty-eight hours before the investigation', she asserted, as she held up the dietary sheet then put it away before I had time to get my glasses out. My options as a vegan were extremely limited – mostly white bread, white pasta, and pealed potatoes, all foods I generally avoid.

Understanding that it could reduce bloating caused by air pumped into the colon during the procedure, I asked, 'Can I take peppermint beforehand?'

'No. Nothing!' she responded, as to a greedy boy who had asked for a second bag of sweeties. 'You can have it afterwards, not before.' She was in no mood for concessions. 'We can sedate you or give you laughing gas', she continued, striking a more conciliatory note.

'Oh, I like laughing gas…' That was much more appealing – even something to look forward to, like sweeties.

*

Three days later it was community night at Sukhavati, and also the date on which my hormone therapy finished. It was twelve weeks exactly since the last shot. From now onwards the drug would slowly leave my system and finally I could recover from my treatments. Everyone was very happy for me when I announced it, and I did not wish to spoil things by mentioning the colonoscopy, even though I was confident of a positive outcome. I also knew I must not take that for granted.

However, the frequency of the bleeding slowly increased; by the time of the colonoscopy it was almost daily. I had also been troubled by mild abdominal pain for weeks before the bleeding had commenced, and I had had the most severe bout of diarrhoea I have ever had outside India. Perhaps inevitably, thoughts about cancer had crept into the dark recesses of my mind.

I did not want to think about it, but I felt impelled as the omens seemed progressively unpropitious; I wanted to be prepared. What would I do if I had bowel cancer? The treatments I had had for prostate cancer had saved my life, but I had long made up my mind not to go through chemo or radiotherapy a second time; surgery was equally unappealing. I do not believe in life at any price and, if diagnosed, would let nature take its course.

Purgatorial

The night before the procedure, I had to take a powerful laxative, drinking litres and litres of water, with a second dose at 6am the following day – an exhausting process, unsettlingly reminiscent of radiotherapy prep. The large intestine needed to be empty for the colonoscopy.

I had my first dose at 7pm as instructed, but, by 10pm, there were no signs of life in my nether regions.

'You've hardly eaten anything for the last couple of days. There's probably nothing in there', said Alex in his soft Northern Irish brogue. His frustrations with the NHS had driven him out of medicine, like quite a few young medics, and he now worked for a firm of stockbrokers in the City. As a former junior registrar surgeon, he was the one member of my community who was familiar with the preparation I was undergoing.

'Ah', I responded, doubtfully. I was convinced that the scrambled eggs and cheese toasties I had been eating as part of my prep had gridlocked my system. Alex, who is sceptical about veganism, seemed amused by my lapse, temporary though it was.

'Look, just drink loads of water', Alex continued. 'That'll clean you out.'

There were minor stirrings after I had gone to bed –

just enough to disrupt my sleep throughout the night, but certainly no Dunkirk-scale evacuation.

'Are you sure this stuff works?', I asked Alex in the morning.

'Oh, it works right enough; it's powerful stuff. Just keep on drinking loads of water', he reiterated. 'It puts downward pressure on the system.' This was no mere theoretical knowledge, but the voice of experience. As junior doctors, he and his mates had spiked each other's drinks with it.

I did as he advised, and before long felt the full impact of purgation. That morning I dared not stray far from the toilet bowl. Had I been sensible I would have decamped to the loo, as I seemed to be spending more time in it than out; then there would have been no risk of a lockout when my legs were driven with preternatural speed to that most private of places – no rapid repetition of 'hang on' resounding in my mind.

I left somewhat nervously for the hospital shortly after midday. I was fearful not of the colonoscopy, but of being stranded, during that interminable fifteen-minute walk, without even a thunderbox nearby. When I finally reached the hospital I was mightily relieved, but still troubled by a tinge of anxiety. The purgation was still in process. Perhaps I had drunk too much water; it seemed to be constantly streaming out.

*

At the endoscopy clinic I was briefed initially by a pretty black nurse whose winning smile at once put me at ease.

Despite my embarrassment, I came clean. 'I'm not sure that I'm completely empty.'

'Is it just fluid?'

'Yes.'

'Oh, that's perfectly normal.'

'But what if it comes out during the procedure?' was the question I could not quite bring myself to ask, but which continued to trouble me.

She conducted me to a changing room where I donned the mandatory, backless NHS gown, so familiar to me from radiotherapy and whose ties I have never yet succeeded in fastening together properly. A few minutes later, there was a knock at the door, then in came a young woman in standard NHS hospital kit.

'I'm the doctor who will be conducting your investigation today', she said, sitting down as a glance of recognition passed between us. 'I think we met in the lift.'

'Indeed, we did', I confirmed, responding immediately to her friendly introduction, before we continued to the briefing.

'I definitely don't want to be sedated', I asserted, once the pleasantries were out of the way, and so we discussed alternatives: a painkiller or the gas – or possibly a combination (if I understood correctly). I was sorely tempted by the gas for dubious reasons, but decided to go ahead without either, as there was more kudos in that. But I was not entirely sure. 'Could I have the gas on standby in case it gets too uncomfortable?'

'Of course, but most people who go without experience minimal discomfort – usually when the scope goes around the bends of the colon.'

We left for the treatment room and I got onto the bed. It was now or never; I had to say it: 'I think I might… leak a bit.'

'There's a reason why we don't treat you in your own clothes', she responded with an amused smile. I chuckled and finally relaxed completely as my curiosity came to the fore.

'How many bends are there?' Not many, but there were ridges and slight twists as the scope explored the alien landscape of my inflated innards whose appearance on the screen above me was reminiscent of scenes from a science-fiction film. I watched, utterly fascinated, as the camera investigated every nook and cranny of my large intestine; my radiographers would have been proud of me – it was completely empty. The sometimes-bizarre sensations, as the camera progressed, or when I had to be turned to face the opposite side, were not at all painful.

The blood and its source were visible from the very beginning. There seemed to be an alarming amount of blood – perhaps because of the enlarged image on the screen – but there were no tumours. I felt a slight pinch as two samples were taken for biopsy from the site of the bleeding, but little else. I was suffering from radiation proctitis – unpleasant, but treatable. Radiotherapy's parting kiss! Recovering from cancer treatment can take a long time. And I wondered whether this would be the final farewell.

'How was my prep?'

'Better side of average.'

'Oh…' Only that? I was a little disappointed.

Then almost suspiciously, 'Do you eat lots of seeds?'

'… Yeeees', a little cautious.

'Thought so', she replied, smiling enigmatically. What was behind that smile – visions of expanding pumpkins and rising sunflowers taking root? Better grind the seeds.

There would be a follow-up consultation with my GP, then a later one in the clinic. But the latter never happened; an uninvited guest had arrived.

By phone

Covid was wreaking havoc across the world, disrupting Western society on an unprecedented scale in my lifetime. Consequently, like many cancer patients, I missed a routine blood test, and the consultation with my oncologist, several weeks after the colonoscopy, was by phone. 'Your blood results have always been excellent; you don't need a test', she assured me. 'I had, in any case, been thinking of switching your reviews from six-monthly to yearly.'

Six months later, even without a test, her registrar informed me that it looked like my cancer was probably cured. But I have no confidence in that word where this uninvited guest is concerned and prefer not to hear it. He arranged a test for me, which showed my PSA to be 0.1.

A further six months passed, and I received a call from the hospital reminding me that I had an appointment the following morning in the hospital.

'Do I?' I responded, surprised. 'I was told it would be a telephone consultation.'

'Oh, didn't you get the notice?'

'No.'

'Sorry about that, but your doctor wants to see you.'

Mask-to-mask

My consultant greeted me with characteristic warmth as I walked into her room. 'It must be eighteen months…' It was. I was very pleased to see her again, even though we were both behind masks.

'I called you in because I had not seen you for so long, and we need to see cancer patients face-to-face', she explained. 'It's not always easy to tell over the phone whether or not people are well.' Perhaps it's not entirely easy even when they are present, but wearing a mask. I could easily understand the importance of meeting patients in person, and had wondered how other cancer patients were managing – how many had been less fortunate than me during the pandemic. I had certainly heard of a few unlucky cases.

'Your PSA is at 0.26', she informed me. 'Hormone therapy keeps your PSA low, but we know that after three years you need no more. It either works or it doesn't', she added starkly. 'PSA then tends to rise slowly until it reaches a certain level.' Because of her mask, I could not fully register her expression, but she seemed to be looking at me as she had done eighteen months before, whether in warning or in reassurance, I could not tell, repeating her words from our previous meeting at the hospital. 'Provided it does not rise above 2, I will not be concerned.'

The routine questions followed until finally she asked, 'Do you have any questions?'

'Yes. Something I have meant to ask for a long time, but kept forgetting.'

'Fire away.'

'Given the particular character of my cancer, had it not been diagnosed when it was, how long would it have taken to metastasize?'

'Oh...' She paused for a moment. 'Difficult to say... You might have been able to sit on it for a few months... but no more. It was caught just in the nick of time.' As I had thought.

There was mention neither of 'cure' nor of twelve-monthly reviews this time, and I was prompted to reflect yet again.

Three years after a chance meeting at the hospital with an acquaintance from the LBC (described in chapter 4), he finally succumbed to his cancer. When we had met, his tumour had just been downgraded from T2 to T1. He had been so relieved, but had shrunk away from me when I told him mine was T3b. Capricious cancer; how ironic that *he* should now be dead while *I* yet live, but I was wary of slipping into complacency. Entertaining cancer is treacherous.

Old age, sickness...

For four years, cancer had forced me to face and reflect upon the deeper realities of life – so often hidden from view in our society; it had exposed my unconscious resistance to seeing what was immediately before me and, indeed, all of us.

We are increasingly shielded from contact with old age, sickness, and death. Our encounters with them tend to be minimal. Old people often pass their final years alone, or in care and nursing homes – we no longer live with them; the seriously ill and dying are mostly dispatched to hospitals – we no longer tend to them; the dead are hidden away in mortuaries and wooden boxes – we no longer keep vigil by them. Thus, we offend the gods, who blind us to the realities of existence, so that, when they impinge upon us, many react with incommensurate fear, are ill-prepared and likely to make bad decisions.

We know that all living things grow old, get sick, and die, but do '*I*' truly understand this will happen to '*me*' (and indeed is already happening)? The less frequently we encounter the stark realities of life, the less likely we are to come to terms with them.

I have grown old and become sick; death is on my horizon, but I am neither morbid nor depressed at the prospect. Facing these facts more fully has enabled me to embrace life far more than had I been imprisoned by overconcern with the seductive mirages of safety and security. If you are prepared to die, you are free to live.

I am approaching the end of a full and deeply satisfying life, with all its struggles, pain, and few triumphs. Though my body is slowly decaying, as decrepitude advances by the year and death becomes progressively alluring, while life stirs in me, I will live as fully as it permits.

Reasons for living...

Shortly after I had completed radiotherapy, a young woman suffering from metastatic breast cancer gave me a book, insisting, 'You must read this; it's my bible.' *Radical Remission*, by Kelly Turner, is essentially an analysis of over a thousand cases of people who had recovered from cancer against all medical expectations. She identifies nine common factors in their recovery, and devotes a chapter to each of them. I was well aware that a bewildering amount of literature and numerous websites are devoted to alternative treatments for cancer, and I was reluctant to read any of them. This was partly because I had already committed myself to a complementary approach to cancer through acupuncture and Chinese medicine with Niccala. After finishing radiotherapy, I had asked Niccala to do whatever she could to help me stay healthy and cancer-free. Naturally she could guarantee nothing, and I certainly had no expectations, but I knew from experience that both she and Jessica had helped me considerably; I had nothing to lose. Nonetheless, I did read Turner's book.

What struck me forcibly was that, of her nine factors, only the first was not already fully part of my life: a radical change to diet. Through Niccala's influence, I was already addressing this, but I then decided to modify my diet much more rigorously. Turner's final factor, 'having strong reasons for living', is something I have in abundance.

... *without a future*

I was in my late twenties, and I had gone to see Bhante. Something was on my mind.

'I'd like to talk about my future', I had said.

'Future? … You don't have a future!' he had responded, chuckling and rendering me speechless. There was nothing else to say. He had hit the mark as surely as the most accomplished Zen master. I had not come for a metaphysical discourse, nor was one necessary.

I had been the driving force behind establishing a Triratna centre in Norwich, and I had become restless and bored; I wanted to move on to something else. He had sensed the restlessness behind my question, and I knew that I must return to my responsibilities with renewed vigour, as I did.

The idea of a future is simply that – a concept; there is no substance to it. In a certain sense, none of us has a future, and yet this non-existent future seduces and distracts us especially when things go wrong, or are particularly uncertain. Therein lies an opportunity. I had had to wait for over seven weeks for confirmation of my cancer diagnosis, and a further four weeks elapsed before I knew for certain that it had not spread. Throughout that period, thoughts about the future had significantly diminished. Consciousness of the uncertainty of my life had focused my mind acutely; my 'future' had been under immediate threat, its vanity exposed – its marked absence was uncannily exhilarating. Once I was convinced that I had a chance of survival, however, the future returned.

We have to think of the future, otherwise we could never plan our lives or achieve very much, but, to do so, while simultaneously comprehending the paradox that there is no future, calls for an understanding well beyond the purely rational and a depth of spiritual insight that I do not yet possess.

*

It is over five years since blood flowed from my penis; had my cancer passed unnoticed much longer, probably I would have been dead by now. But I am alive and, despite my age, I have so much to live for.

Within Triratna, those who have requested ordination may ask two Order members to be their kalyana mitras, or spiritual friends; though Matt was only twenty-three, he asked me to be one of his. I was delighted, but apparently I had replied, 'Okay, provided you fix us with at least three gigs a year.' My conditional response was not serious, but he took me at my word and had quickly arranged our next two 'poetry and jazz' gigs.

I am constantly revived by youth – not my own long-fled early years, of course, but by the stimulus of my many young friends. Years ago, I had realized that I needed the company of young people; they rejuvenate me, but not in a vicarious way. Their zest for life, optimism, and idealism are catalysts for revitalizing those same qualities in me. They have helped to steer me away from the bitterness and cynicism that so often mar the later years of older people, without diminishing the experience that has formed me; I have always tried to learn from the vicissitudes of life. I am also conscious that, just as I need young people, they need contact with the experience of those who have made a life-long effort to become a better and still better human being.

I live in a building on a busy road in London, very close to a police station and a fire station, at a junction controlled by traffic lights. Sirens scream throughout the night, almost constantly at weekends. It is not the most restful environment, but I also live in a community with eleven other men, none of whom is over thirty-five, and there is nowhere else I would rather be. Youth is the perfect tonic for an old man with cancer.

No story is ever finished until the protagonist ceases to be. My story, like all stories, can only truly end with my inevitable death – which is probably not far off. But that is a conclusion I cannot write, and so this will have to serve in its stead. I am currently in remission from cancer, and that is now all I can tell you. If I am lucky, I will remain so long enough to die of something else.

Notes and References

1   John Keats, as recorded by his friend Charles Armitage Brown in
    The Life of John Keats, Oxford University Press, London 1937, p.64,
    widely quoted by Keats' biographers.

2   *The Hundred Thousand Songs of Milarepa*, trans. Garma C.C.
    Chang, Shambhala, London and Boulder, CO, 1977, pp.111, 129,
    131, 132, 142, 212.

3   *Alastor, or The Spirit of Solitude*, in *The Poetical Works of Shelley*,
    Oxford University Press, London 1912, p.28, lines 639–40.

4   Santideva, *Entering the Path of Enlightenment*, trans. Marion Matics,
    Allen & Unwin, London 1971, p.153.

5   William Shakespeare, Sonnet 73, in *William Shakespeare: The
    Complete Works*, Collins, London and Glasgow 1951, p.1320.

6   D.H. Lawrence, *The Ship of Death*, in *The Complete Poems of D.H.
    Lawrence*, Penguin, Harmondsworth 1977, p.720, section X, lines
    105–7.

7   William Shakespeare, *Cymbeline*, in *William Shakespeare: The
    Complete Works*, p.1225, act 4, scene 2, lines 259–60.

8   John Donne, *Meditation XVII: Devotions upon Emergent Occasions
    and Death's Duel*, Vintage, New York 1999, pp.102–3.

WINDHORSE PUBLICATIONS

Windhorse Publications is a Buddhist charitable company based in the United Kingdom. We place great emphasis on producing books of high quality that are accessible and relevant to those interested in Buddhism at whatever level. We are the main publisher of the works of Sangharakshita, the founder of the Triratna Buddhist Order and Community. Our books draw on the whole range of the Buddhist tradition, including translations of traditional texts, commentaries, books that make links with contemporary culture and ways of life, biographies of Buddhists, and works on meditation.

As a not-for-profit enterprise, we ensure that all surplus income is invested in new books and improved production methods, to better communicate Buddhism in the twenty-first century. We welcome donations to help us continue our work – to find out more, go to windhorsepublications.com.

The Windhorse is a mythical animal that flies over the earth carrying on its back three precious jewels, bringing these invaluable gifts to all humanity: the Buddha (the 'awakened one'), his teaching, and the community of all his followers.

Windhorse Publications
38 Newmarket Road
Cambridge CB5 8DT
info@windhorsepublications.com

Consortium Book Sales & Distribution
210 American Drive
Jackson TN 38301
USA

Windhorse Books
PO Box 574
Newtown NSW 2042
Australia

THE TRIRATNA BUDDHIST COMMUNITY

Windhorse Publications is a part of the Triratna Buddhist Community, an international movement with centres in Europe, India, North and South America, and Australasia. At these centres, members of the Triratna Buddhist Order offer classes in meditation and Buddhism. Activities of the Triratna Community also include retreat centres, residential spiritual communities, ethical Right Livelihood businesses, and the Karuna Trust, a United Kingdom fundraising charity that supports social welfare projects in the slums and villages of India.

Through these and other activities, Triratna is developing a unique approach to Buddhism, not simply as a philosophy and a set of techniques, but as a creatively directed way of life for all people living in the conditions of the modern world.

If you would like more information about Triratna please visit thebuddhistcentre.com or write to:

London Buddhist Centre
51 Roman Road
London E2 0HU
United Kingdom

Aryaloka
14 Heartwood Circle
Newmarket NH 03857
USA

Sydney Buddhist Centre
24 Enmore Road
Sydney NSW 2042
Australia

It's Not Out There: How to See Differently and Live an Extraordinary, Ordinary Life

Danapriya

Most of us constantly look outside ourselves for something: happiness, love, contentment. But this something is not out there. 'It' is within us. We are full of these qualities: happiness, love, contentment and more.

In *It's Not Out There*, Buddhist teacher and mentor, Danapriya, helps you to look inside yourself in such a way that life becomes more vivid, joyful and extraordinary.

If you want to suffer less and to live life more fully, this book is for you. It's about seeing the reality of the human predicament, and seeing through the illusions that create unnecessary pain for yourself and others. This book uncovers the fertile ground of your own potential, and enables you to live the life you are here for. Stop, look, listen and sense, you are worth it.

Written in simple, down-to-earth language, It's Not Out There *is brimming with practical wisdom. Positive and encouraging, Danapriya shares ways to help anyone who wants to change their life and find greater happiness and fulfilment.* – Dr Paramabandhu Groves, co-author of *Eight Step Recovery: Using the Buddha's Teachings to Overcome Addiction*

Reading this book is like having a conversation with a wise friend – someone who doesn't just talk at you but who is interested in your thoughts and experience too. Buy one for everyone you know who is serious about life and how to live it well. – Subhadramati, author of *Not About Being Good*

Born Ian Dixon in 1959, Danapriya ('one who loves giving') has been involved in personal growth and healing work for over three decades. Ordained into the Triratna Buddhist Order in 2001, he founded the Deal Buddhist Group in Kent, UK, in 2007. Based there, he continues to lead retreats and teach meditation, while also running the counselling business *Talking Listening Clarity*. www.danapriya.org

ISBN 978-1-911407-59-1
£9.99/$13.95/€11.95
160 pages

Introducing Mindfulness: Buddhist Background and Practical Exercises

Bhikkhu Anālayo

Buddhist meditator and scholar Bhikkhu Anālayo introduces the Buddhist background to mindfulness practice, from mindful eating to its formal cultivation as *satipaṭṭhāna* (the foundations of mindfulness). As well as providing an accessible guide, Anālayo gives a succinct historical survey of the development of mindfulness in Buddhism, and practical exercises on how to develop it.

A wise and helpful presentation of essential elements of the Buddha's teaching . . . it will be of great value for those who wish to put these teachings into practice. A wonderful Dharma gift. – Joseph Goldstein, author of *Mindfulness: A Practical Guide to Awakening*

A gold mine for anyone who is working in the broad field of mindfulness-based programs for addressing health and wellbeing in the face of suffering – in any or all of its guises. – Jon Kabat-Zinn, author of *Meditation Is Not What You Think: Mindfulness and Why It Is So Important*

Bhikkhu Anālayo offers simple skilled mindfulness practices for each of the dimensions of this book. Open-minded practices of embodied mindfulness are described, beginning with eating and health, and continuing with mindfulness examining mind and body, our relation to death, and the nature of the mind itself. Significantly, by highlighting the earliest teachings on internal and external mindfulness, Bhikkhu Anālayo shows how, individually and collectively, we can use mindfulness to bring a liberating understanding to ourselves and to the pressing problems of our global, social, modern world. We need this more than ever. – Jack Kornfield, from the Foreword

ISBN 978 1 911407 57 7
£13.99/$18.95/€16.95
176 pages

A Deeper Beauty: Buddhist Reflections on Everyday Life

Paramananda

The best-selling author of *Change Your Mind* suggests ways of uncovering meaning, depth and stillness in lives often fuelled by activity and bombarded with information. Using reflections and stories from his own life, he discusses themes such as poetry, death, joy and imagination, offering courage and kindness in the search for meaning.

ISBN 9781 899579 44 0
£10.99/$16.95/€13.95
208 pages

Buddhism: Tools for Living Your Life

Vajragupta

In this guide for all those seeking a meaningful spiritual path, Vajragupta provides clear explanations of the main Buddhist teachings, as well as a variety of exercises designed to help readers develop or deepen their practice.

Appealing, readable, and practical, blending accessible teachings, practices, and personal stories . . . as directly relevant to modern life as it is comprehensive and rigorous. – Tricycle: The Buddhist Review, 2007

I'm very pleased that someone has finally written this book! At last, a real 'toolkit' for living a Buddhist life, his practical suggestions are hard to resist! – Saddhanandi, Director of Adhisthana

ISBN 9781 899579 74 7
£12.99/$18.95/€17.95
192 pages

CPSIA information can be obtained
at www.ICGtesting.com
Printed in the USA
JSHW042345181221
21378JS00004B/5